The Caregiver's Guide to Self-Care

Help for Your Caregiving Journey

By
Jane Meier Hamilton, MSN, RN

ARPress
ILLUMINATING IDEAS
EMPOWERING VOICES

ARPress LLC
45 Dan Road Suite 5
Canton MA 02021
Hotline: 1(888) 821-0229
Fax: 1(508) 545-7580

Ordering Information:
Quantity sales. Special discounts are available on quantity purchases by corporations, associations, and others. For details, contact the publisher at the address above.

Printed in the United States of America.

ISBN-13:   Softcover   979-8-89330-407-7
           Hardcover   979-8-89330-409-1
           eBook   979-8-89330-408-4

Library of Congress Control Number: 2024901190

TABLE OF CONTENTS

- o Environmental Strategies: Draw energy from your home, imagination and nature
- o Psychological Strategies: Use your mind and mindfulness practices
- o Social Strategies: Reach out and connect with others
- o Spiritual Strategies: Reflect, connect and give thanks
- o Family Strategies: Cultivate the qualities of resilient families
- Activities for Caregivers
- Helpful Resources

PREFACE

Your loved one needs your help and you are doing the very best you can. Some days helping them feels great. When you think of how much they mean to you, how much they have given, or how vulnerable they are, you throw yourself into caregiving.

But at other times, caring for your loved one can be overwhelming and burdensome. So much of your own life is put on hold. So much of your energy and resources are spent. And your heart can be utterly broken by the pain and suffering you witness. If you withdraw or turn away, guilt rises; you wonder how you could react this way. But these mixed feelings are normal, human. Caring for another person is never easy. At times it is terribly difficult and painful, almost unbearable. Being a caregiver can make you sick in body, mind and spirit. And this is why I wrote *The Caregiver's Guide to Self-Care: Help for Your Caregiving Journey.*

My caregiving journey spans many years. I have been a registered nurse for over 40 years and a family caregiver for 20. Although caring for others has been meaningful and fulfilling—it has not always been easy. Being a nurse was physically, mentally, and emotionally demanding work. But accompanying those I love through pain and severe illness challenged me on a much deeper level. Caring for my husband, my parents, in-laws and friends, touched my heart and soul in profound ways that changed me and called me into my current work, caring for caregivers. Easing the burden of caregiver stress and equipping caregivers for their journey has become my mission.

The key lesson I took from my caregiving experience is this: ***All of us who give care need to take care.*** If we overlook our own needs, our physical and mental health suffers. We begin to feel alone, overwhelmed and become unable to effectively help those in our care. These things happened to me.

Many times I was overwhelmed by caregiving, but I discovered things that relieved my stress, protected my health, and sustained my capacity to care. These are the ideas that you'll find in this 2ⁿᵈ edition of *The Caregiver's Guide to Self-Care*. The model I first published in 2011, "The 7C's of Self-Care" offered seven strategies that worked for me, and was consistent with other evidence-based, wellness models.

Over the years, I've refined my model, integrating current research on caregiving, positive psychology, and resilience. This 2ⁿᵈ edition presents new concepts, recommendations, activities and resources that I'm sure you'll find helpful. In each chapter you will find:

- ***Jane's Story*** a brief, personal reflection on my own experience as a daughter struggling to cope with my mother's dementia.

- ***Self-care Recommendations*** from my professional experience as a psychiatric nurse that are based on research from the stress, caregiving, and positive psychology literature.

- ***Activities for Caregivers*** to help individual caregivers, groups of caregivers, or professionals who are helping caregivers. These are designed to guide you in applying self-care concepts in your life. Read through them all; focus on those that work for you.

- ***Helpful Resources*** that provide additional information about caregiving and self-care for caregivers, as well as some inspiring quotes.

Your loved one needs your help and you are doing the very best you can in one of life's most important and challenging jobs. To "go the distance" on your caregiving journey, ***care for yourself as you care for*** *others*. My earnest hope is that you find compassion, comfort and real help in this 2nd edition of *The Caregiver's Guide to Self-Care: Help for Your Caregiving Journey*. Thank you for allowing me to join you on your caregiving journey....

Jane Meier Hamilton, MSN, RN
May, 2022

CHAPTER 1

Caregivers and Caregiving

We all know about the 18 million *professional caregivers* who are part of the "paid" healthcare workforce: doctors, nurses, nursing assistants, companions, to name a few. But do you know there are over 53 million *family caregivers* in America; roughly one-third of all adults and all households in the US?

Family caregivers are women and men who care for a loved one who is ill, disabled, elderly or a special-needs child. They care without pay and often without any training. They are people of any age, race or sex; of any financial, religious, employment or socio-economic group.

There is not a family in America that isn't impacted by caregiving, at one time or another. In the words of former First Lady, Rosalynn Carter, "There are only four kinds of people in the world: those who <u>have been</u> caregivers, those who <u>currently are</u> caregivers, those who <u>will be</u> caregivers and those who <u>will need</u> caregivers." *Caregiving is a universal experience.*

What Every Caregiver Experiences

Embedded within this universal experience there are six common characteristics that every caregiver experiences.

1. **A Story**: There is another well-known saying, "When you've seen one caregiver, you've seen one caregiver."

   While caregiving touches everyone's life, caregiving is an individual experience. *All caregivers have a personal story that is uniquely their own.* Who is the care receiver and what is their relationship to the caregiver? What is their condition and its prognosis? What is the nature of care required and how does this impact on the caregiver's personal and work life?

   No two stories are alike but there are universal components to those stories, as described by these six characteristics listed here. Also, like any other story, caregiving stories have a beginning, middle and end; caregivers journey through the story. Caregiving stories evolve over time. Characters change and often grow as the story progresses. There can be moments of high drama and periods of dullness or even boredom. *Every caregiver has their unique story.*

2. **Stressors**: Stressors are the demands of life that cause stress. There are two types of stressors that all caregivers encounter. First, there are the *caregiving tasks* that must be done. Second are *personal caregiving challenges*. These are individually felt, often deep and powerful internal feelings that caregivers experience. Though invisible to others, challenges like these can cause a great deal of stress for caregivers. *Every caregiver encounters stressors that cause stress.*

3. **A Toll**: On average, the caregiving journey lasts 4.6 years; a third provide care for more than 5 years. It exposes caregivers to varying degrees of chronic stress which can erode a caregiver's health, well-being and capacity to care; 60% report moderate to significant decline in their own health. The nature of the toll varies from person to person. *Caregiving takes some kind of a toll on every caregiver.*

4. **Needs**: It is not only the care receiver who has needs. Every caregiver has their own needs which must be met as they journey through caregiving. These are: *A) Practical, problem-solving help; B) Positive personal energy; and C) Partners in providing care.* Like their story, caregivers' needs are felt in uniquely personal ways. *Every caregiver must attend to their own needs.*

5. **Self-Care**: Not simply something "nice-to-do," s*elf-care is a necessity* for preserving a caregiver's well-being and capacity to care. It's important that caregivers *admit* their need for self-care; *permit* themselves the time for self-care; and *commit* to regularly practicing healthy self-care. This includes healthy practices that nurture the body, mind and emotions; anything spiritual, social or fun-loving that connects them with others. *Healthy self-care practices are tailored to each caregiver's preferences*; whatever healthy behavior brings them joy, relaxation, calm or peace. *Every caregiver requires self-care.*

6. **A Relay**: Because caregiving journeys are often long and challenging, they are too big to handle alone. Envisioning a race, caregiving is *not a sprint* which is quickly finished. It's *not a marathon* that is run using the energy of only one person. Caregiving is like a *relay*, a race with multiple heats run by numerous runners who work as a team and pass the baton from person to person. Each runs their own leg of the race and all rely on each other to "go the distance" and finish the race. *Every caregivers needs to collaborate with care partners.*

Physical, Emotional, and Financial Impact of Caregiving

Over 25 years of research have documented how *caregiving impacts the physical, emotional, and financial health of caregivers.* Compared with the general population, caregivers face greater ***physical*** health risks:

- Minor ailments like headache, muscle strain, or upset stomach
- Major ailments like heart disease, diabetes, arthritis or cancer

- Greater risk of falls for older adult caregivers
- Sleep disturbances
- Weight changes

Caregivers are twice as likely as non-caregivers to have significant chronic conditions like heart disease, diabetes, arthritis, or cancer. And chronic stress can take as many as ten years off their lives. Health differences are more pronounced for Millennial caregivers, than for those who are members of Gen X, Baby Boomers, or communities of color.

The *emotional* effect of caregiving can be significant. Between 40-70% of caregivers report moderate to severe depression; one-third report moderate to severe anxiety. Caregivers use prescriptions medications for depression and anxiety at 2-3 times the rate of the general population.

Nearly a quarter (21%) of caregivers report loneliness. In those who describe "feeling alone," 72% report high levels of emotional distress. The **Burden Scale for Family Caregivers** measures the intensity of the strain experienced as a result of caregiving. A higher score, reflects a greater impact on caregiver well-being and health. (Check out your level of caregiver burden using the questionnaire found in Chapter 4: *The Toll Self-Care Activity #1: Is my health "at risk" because of caregiving?*)

Negative physical and emotional consequences aren't inevitable; 44% of spousal caregivers report no strain. Many caregivers don't report high stress; they cope successfully, and get positive psychological benefits from providing care to loved ones.

Finally, caregiving can also significantly affect *financial* health. One in five caregivers report high financial strain due to caregiving. Nearly half experience at least one financial impact: assuming debt, borrowing money, not paying bills or paying late, stopping savings or using up savings on caregiving expenses. More than two-thirds of caregivers provide some financial support to their care receiver. On average, caregivers spend $10,000/year out-of-pocket on caregiving-related costs.

Staying Well Throughout the Caregiving Journey

Given these facts about the impact of caregiving, it's clear that healthy self-care is of critical importance. In the following chapters, you'll find evidence-based information, activities and advice on *how to stay well all along the caregiving journey.* These proven and practical self-care practices are not difficult. Use the stories, text, recommendations, and activities to discover ways to care for yourself as you care for others. It will be good for you and for the one in your care.

CHAPTER 2

Caregiver Stories: Universal and Uniquely Personal

Jane's Story: There is a Season and a Time

I have been a caregiver many times during the past twenty years. Many members of my immediate and extended family have needed my help as they battled a host of serious illnesses. And I am not alone in this. Many of my close friends have cared for their spouses, parents and children, too. In some cases, those we love have died, but others now live with chronic conditions that have forever changed their lives. Seeing family and friends suffer has broken my heart and created within me a deep desire to help.

For me, the desire and ability to care for my loved ones was like a precious pearl, secreted away deep inside me. Our bonds of affection created this pearl of great price. When their days of need arrived, I reached deep within to where the pearl was hidden. Out of love and compassion I redeemed that treasure and spent all its worth to provide for them. Because I have felt their love, I wanted to return it with helpful, caring acts. This is how I became a caregiver. The time of my loved ones' need became my season of care.

To everything there is a season and a time to every purpose under heaven. Is this your season of care? Is this your time to help a loved one? Is it your purpose to be a caregiver? Many people don't think of themselves as caregivers. They say,

- "I am his wife, not a caregiver."
- "She's my mother; after all she's done for me, it's the least I can do."
- "I am just helping my friend; I want to be there for him."
- "I never thought of myself as a caregiver; I just do things for my Dad."
- "We're family; it's no big deal."

Sometimes *it is* a big deal, though, even with the desire and ability to care. Occasionally it is a debt or duty, not voluntarily chosen. Caring for a loved one is not the same as being a paid or professional caregiver. At its best, family caregiving is not employment; it is a testament to, and a repayment of love.

Are you a family caregiver? If so, recognize the wonderful gifts you give. *Claim your caregiver role.*

Self-Care Recommendations

What do you mean by "caregiver"?

Within our families, neighborhoods, faith communities, workplaces, health care practices and circles of friends, we know people of all ages who are caring for loved ones. Today, in any given year over 53 million people in the US provide care for a chronically ill, disabled or aged family member, or special needs child. Based on demographic trends, these numbers are sure to rise in the years ahead. Many of these millions don't think of themselves as caregivers. They see themselves not heroes but as helpers, who are looking to give back, not get recognition.

When referring to caregivers, several terms are used.

- *Professional caregivers* are the paid workers or unpaid volunteers who work in health care organizations, faith-based, or community organizations.

- *Family caregivers* are unpaid individuals who take care of their family members, friends or neighbors. They provide many types of care: emotional support, physical care and help managing household or personal affairs. The amount of time spent on family caregiving can range from a few hours a week to round the clock responsibility.

- *Primary caregivers* actually deliver care. Those providing hands-on help can be either a professional, family member or friend.

- *Secondary caregivers* act as backup support to primary caregivers, those family members or professionals who provide direct care.

- *Long-distance caregivers* are family caregivers who live more than an hour's travel distance from a care receiver.

You may recognize yourself, or someone you know, in these descriptions. Like others, you may not usually think of yourself in these terms, even though you do provide support for a loved one…caring is just something you do! But when providing care, it is important to identify yourself as a caregiver with important needs. Why?

- Providing ongoing care and assistance can take a physical, financial, emotional and spiritual toll.

- Caregiving can strain your work life and family relations.

- Overlooking the impact of caregiving puts you at risk of feeling isolated, overwhelmed, and becoming ill.

- Support from others and your our own self-care can help you stay healthy and strong enough to do one of the most important things you will ever do in life…and that's good for both you and the one in your care.

So, if you or someone you know is a family caregiver, review these materials. You may have little free time but you owe it to yourself to invest some time to find resources and people who can help you. You are not alone. The first steps to receiving the support you need are recognizing your role as caregiver, and the stress that often comes with it.

Activities for Caregivers

Caregiver Stories Self-Care Activity #1: Am I a caregiver?

Caregiving Role Questionnaire					
You may not think of yourself as a caregiver; even though you do a lot to help your loved one…it's just something you do! Check the four ways that caregivers typically offer help to family and friends. If you assist in any of these ways, yes, you are a family caregiver.					
Read the statements below. Circle the number that best describes your experience:	Constantly	Very often	With some regularity	Very rarely	Never
A. I provide physical care: feed, bathe, dress, groom, toilet, or help with walking.	4	3	2	1	0
B. I manage household affairs: cook, clean, shop, launder clothes, do home repairs, or help with relocation.	4	3	2	1	0
C. I manage personal affairs: medicine, finances, legal, insurance, care coordination, or transportation.	4	3	2	1	0
D. I provide emotional or social support: help with behavior, moods, socializing, or making decisions.	4	3	2	1	0
Scoring: Add-up the numbers you circled. To interpret your score, see the **Interpreting My Score** guide below.	**My score is:** _____				

©Partners on the Path. 2022. www.PartnersonthePath.com

Caregiver Stories Self-Care Activity #1: Interpreting My Score

Items with a score of 3 or 4 are areas where you are heavily involved. Regardless of your composite score, these responsibilities require energy and are demanding.

Any total score above 4 indicates that you have taken on a family caregiving role. Thinking of yourself as a caregiver is important because it opens your eyes to the:

- Beautiful gift you give when helping others in need.
- Toll that caregiving can take on you.
- Need to protect your health, well-being and capacity to care.

Total scores of 1-7 suggest that you are not burdened by caregiving at this time.

Total scores of 8-16 reveal that you have significant caregiving responsibilities. Though these may be very meaningful to you, they may erode your well-being and health, particularly if you have been a caregiver for a long time, or in difficult situations. Protect yourself. Take care.

Higher numbers suggest the need to focus on self-care because you may be vulnerable to the effects of caregiver stress. Any of these scores can change over time, so check yourself again in the future, as a way to keep aware of your situation.

Caregiver Stories Self-Care Activity #2: What stage of caregiving am I in?

<table>
<tr>
<td colspan="3"><u>Stage of Caregiving Checklist</u>

Caregiving is a journey with a series of different stages along the way. As a caregiver, what you do and how you feel changes over time. Where are you on the caregiving path?

Directions: Review each of the stages. Check the stage that best describes your current caregiving experience.</td>
</tr>
<tr>
<td>_____</td>
<td>Stage 1: Preparing Myself
Approaching the path
Caring for my loved one is in my future.</td>
<td>Typical Stage 1 experiences:
Observing growing needs in your loved one
Thinking they may soon need your help
Feeling: Surprise, concern about changes you see
Wondering: What lies ahead? Where can I turn for information?</td>
</tr>
<tr>
<td>_____</td>
<td>Stage 2: Getting Started
Entering onto the path
I am starting to care for my loved one.</td>
<td>Typical Stage 2 experiences:
Offering various types of help
Seeing how caregiving fits with your other roles
Learning about the condition, helpful resources
Feeling: Denial, fear, confusion, sadness, hopefulness
Wondering: What is happening? Why?</td>
</tr>
<tr>
<td>_____</td>
<td>Stage 3: Actively Helping
Walking the path
I am offering care to my loved one.</td>
<td>Typical Stage 3 experiences:
Helping regularly, for a number of months or years
Assuring your loved one's growing needs are met
Coordinating with others to offer help
Feeling: Ambivalence, satisfaction, frustration, fatigue, sadness
Wondering: What needs to be done? How will we do it?</td>
</tr>
<tr>
<td>_____</td>
<td>Stage 4: Struggling Along
Staggering along the path
My caregiving continues and it's hard.</td>
<td>Typical Stage 4 experiences:
Providing increasingly heavy level of care
Adjusting to your loved one's change/decline
Needing support to continue helping
Feeling: Resentment, guilt, anger, exhaustion, overwhelmed
Wondering: How long can this go on? How long can I go on?</td>
</tr>
</table>

	Stage 5: Letting Go Nearing the end of the path Caregiving as I know it is ending.	**Typical Stage 5 experiences:** Preparing to change your role as caregiver Facing loved one's end-of-life or "new normal" Considering quality of life vs. longevity Forgiving yourself and others **Feeling:** Loss, release, powerlessness, introspective **Wondering:** Is this really happening?
	Stage 6: Moving On Leaving the path I am no longer a caregiver.	**Typical Stage 6 experiences:** Mourning Reflecting on the lessons and meaning of caregiving Sharing your wisdom Considering your future **Feeling:** Grief, pride, relief, regret, return of energy **Wondering:** What does the future hold for me?

Caregiver Stories Self-Care Activity #3: Guided Self-Reflection

<u>**My Caregiving Story: Guided Self-Reflection**</u>
<u>Directions</u>: To help you put things in perspective, think about important elements of your caregiving story by responding to the following questions.

1.	**What's good about it?**

<u>**Name It**</u>
- What are the good parts of caring for my loved one?
- What gives me a sense of joy or happiness?
- What is meaningful to me or to my loved one?
- What am I proudest of doing?
- What is important about my being a caregiver?

2.	**What's not so good about it?**

<u>**Name It**</u>
- What are the most difficult parts of caring for my loved one?
- What brings me sorrow or pain?
- What is frustrating or annoying about this role?
- How do these difficulties, sorrows or frustrations affect me?

3.	What are positive outcomes from my caregiving journey?
Name It • What lessons have I learned from being a caregiver? • How have I grown or changed as a result of caring for my loved one? • How has being a caregiver enriched my life?	

©Partners on the Path. 2022. www.PartnersonthePath.com

Helpful Resources

Caring for the Caregiver: Claim your caregiver role https://www.youtube.com/watch?v=fYZT8CpT1oo YouTube video of the author describing the importance of claiming your caregiver role.

Family Caregiver Alliance: www.caregiver.org is a national non-profit that has supported and championed the cause of family caregivers for over 40 years. Their highly regarded care management offerings include:

- Caregiver Education Resources by Health Issue or Condition: https://www.caregiver.org/caregiver-resources/health-conditions/

- Online Support Groups: https://www.caregiver.org/connecting-caregivers/support-groups/

Green, Eboni Ivory. *Caregiving in the New Millennium: A Survival Guide for Today's Caregiver. 3ʳᵈ Edition.* Create Space. 2017.

Lunden, Joan and Newmark, Amy. *Chicken Soup for the Soul: Family Caregivers—101 Stories of Love, Sacrifice, and Bonding.* Chicken Soup for the Soul Publishers. 2012.

Powerful Tools for Caregivers: https://www.powerfultoolsforcaregivers.org/ is a highly respected self-care education program for family caregivers that is presented by community-based organizations across the US. Research shows that the 6-week course improves caregivers' wellbeing and effectiveness. Program text, The Caregiver Helpbook, is available in English and Spanish: https://www.powerfultoolsforcaregivers.org/product-category/caregiver-helpbook/

"It's only natural to feel overwhelmed by the prospect of adding caregiving to an already full plate. Ambivalence toward caregiving should be considered a normal, expectable reaction that doesn't invalidate your love or devotion to your ill family member."
Dr. Barry Jacobs
Psychologist and author of *The Emotional Survival Guide for Caregivers*

"Humans think in stories, and we try to make sense of the world by telling stories."
Yuval Noah Harari
Israeli historian and author

"What makes caregiving appear difficult is the inner journey, the one that requires us to summon the courage and flexibility to relate to life in an unfamiliar but more expansive way...Caregiving has heart and meaning because it changes us for the better."
Beth Witrogen McLeod
Speaker and author of *Caregiving: The Spiritual Journey of Love, Loss and Renewal*

CHAPTER 3

Stressors: Causes of Caregiver Stress

Jane's Story: Lost in the Line of Duty

Just this morning, I had a startling realization: I am lost! I usually know where I am going, and I generally reach my goal. But for the first time, I see that I am lost, not in a geographical sense, but in other different and disturbing ways. I have lost my zest for life; my energy is low and I am grief-stricken about Mother's dementia. I have lost my confidence about the future; I have no idea where this disease will take Mom and the rest of us, too. I am often lost in thought, preoccupied with how to get everything done and keep all the balls in the air. I have lost important parts of my life: my image of my parents as strong, vibrant people; my illusions of immortality and invulnerability; my hope that good people will be spared suffering; my sense of being someone's child.

In giving of myself to help my parents, I have lost parts of myself. What are the costs of trading off parts of my life over an extended period of time? What are the benefits? What choices do I have? I am betting that I won't always be lost. I want to help because Mom and Dad won't always need me as they do now. I am gambling that important parts of me can be revived. I hope I am right.

Where are you on your caregiving journey?

When I wrote *Lost in the Line of Duty* I was just waking up to the fact that caring for my parents had become a chronic source of stress. It was beginning to take a toll and I was starting to see my need for help. What had begun as a natural desire to give something back to my parents had silently morphed. Unbeknownst to me, I had become a caregiver. I was beginning to notice other caregivers, many who were doing much, much more than I was. That gave me hope. If they could manage, so could I. The people or diagnoses in your circumstances may be different than mine, but like me you are a caregiver. Where are you on your caregiving journey? Are you lost in the line of duty? What might be the costs and benefits of trading off parts of your life over an extended period of time? Though meaningful, caregiving is stressful and can take a toll on your physical and mental health. Explore the facts about caregiver stress found in this chapter and the many self-care suggestions found throughout this book. These ideas can strengthen you and help preserve your capacity to care.

Self-Care Recommendations

Why do I need to understand caregiver stress?

Though it can be deeply rewarding, giving care is not easy; over time, it can make you sick. Family caregivers face a litany of challenges: physical demands, financial pressures, emotional ups and downs, major changes in roles and responsibilities, unfamiliar patient care duties, and worries about a loved one's welfare, 24/7.

When caregiving goes on for a long time, it erodes your immune system and increases your susceptibility to disease; it increases your risk for depression and hospitalization. About 20-30% of family caregivers suffer from psychological and mood disturbances. Caregivers use prescription drugs for depression, anxiety, and insomnia two to three times as often as the rest of the population. *For your own health and quality of life, it is important that you understand and learn to handle caregiver stress.*

What is caregiver stress?

Life's demands, called stressors, cause stress. Stress is how the body responds to stressors. *Caregiver stress is how you respond to the demands of being a caregiver.* When viewed positively, the demands of caregiving are rewarding or challenging, and actually give you positive energy, but when experienced as negative, caregiver stressors create wear and tear on your body, mind and spirit. Whether your perceptions are positive or negative, *the stress response is a self-protective, 3-phase process of adaptation that safeguards you and keeps you alive.* The nature of your adaptation changes during each phase of the stress response, diagrammed below. No matter how different, each phase of the stress response is protective.

Three Phases of the Stress Response

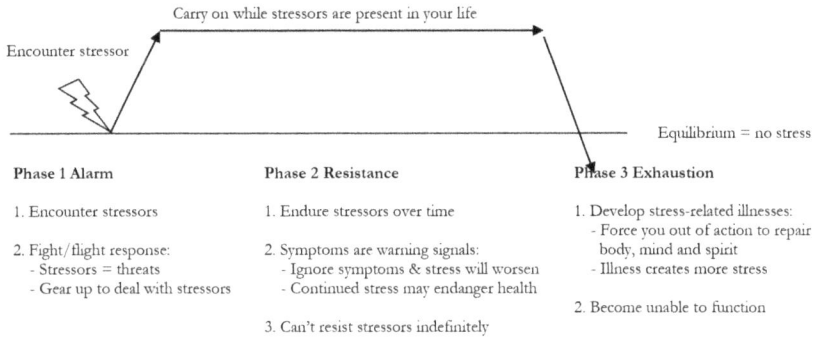

Carry on while stressors are present in your life

Encounter stressor

Equilibrium = no stress

Phase 1 Alarm	Phase 2 Resistance	Phase 3 Exhaustion
1. Encounter stressors	1. Endure stressors over time	1. Develop stress-related illnesses: - Force you out of action to repair body, mind and spirit - Illness creates more stress
2. Fight/flight response: - Stressors = threats - Gear up to deal with stressors	2. Symptoms are warning signals: - Ignore symptoms & stress will worsen - Continued stress may endanger health	2. Become unable to function
	3. Can't resist stressors indefinitely	

Caregiver stress, your health, and the quality and length of your life are all tied together, so it is very important to learn how to handle stress effectively. You have only one body and one life to live. In addition to interfering with your health, mismanaged stress also interferes with your work life, personal life and caregiving relationships. *Using effective stress management techniques protects you from some of these negative effects of stress.*

What are symptoms and sources of caregiver stress?

Recognizing stress in your life requires assessment of two key factors: the symptoms and the sources of stress.

The *symptoms of stress are* your body's way of signaling that you are endangering yourself by remaining in contact with stressors. Symptoms occur while you are in the resistance phase of stress. They foreshadow the illness or burnout that occurs during the exhaustion phase.

Stress symptoms are grouped into *six categories–physical, emotional, mental, social, occupational and spiritual.* Everyone manifests symptoms of stress in each of these six categories, but because every human being is unique, each person experiences their own distinct set of symptoms. Assess your symptoms using the *Stressors Self-Care Activity #1: What are my symptoms of caregiver stress?*

Stressors are life's challenges and demands that cause stress. Some come from within you, while others come from your relationship with the environment and people around you.

- *Internal stressors* are the physical aspects of your own body, the emotions you experience or the demands which you place on yourself.

- *External stressors* arise from physical aspects of your environment—a wide range of factors like storms, traffic jams, power outages, crowded or dirty living arrangements. They also come from the needs, expectations and behaviors of other people.

Every human being experiences a mix of internal and external stressors every day.

As a caregiver, you deal with specific, caregiving-related stressors. Some *common caregiver stressors* are listed in two activities that follow:

- *Stressors Self-Care Activity #2: Why am I so stressed?*
- *Stressors Self-Care Activity #3: What kind of help do I need?*

When you have identified your symptoms and sources of caregiver stress, proceed to the following chapters which will show you practical ways to care for yourself as you care for others.

Activities for Caregivers

Stressors Self-Care Activity #1: What are my symptoms of caregiver stress?

Stress Symptoms Checklist
It is important to be aware of stress symptoms; left unchecked, they lead to stress-related illnesses. Make a check on the line next to any of the caregiver stress symptoms you experience.

Physical

-- Change in appetite	-- Hyperventilation	-- Restlessness
-- Change in weight	-- Trembling	-- Chronic fatigue
-- Eating junk food	-- Muscle tension	-- Insomnia
-- Heavy drinking	-- Teeth grinding	-- Nightmares
-- Smoking	-- Nail biting	-- Headache
-- Drug abuse	-- Clumsiness	-- Sexual difficulties
-- Stomach problems	-- Stooped posture	

Emotional

-- Complaining	-- Mood swings	-- Vulnerability
-- Crying	-- Depression	-- Fear
-- Guilt or shame	-- Apathy	-- Frustration
-- Irritability	-- Inability to feel or express emotions	-- Anger
-- Mistrust	-- Grief or loss	-- Loneliness
-- Anxiety or panic		

Mental

-- Indecisiveness	-- Wishing to return to life as it was before caregiving	-- Boredom
-- Difficulty concentrating		-- Confusion
-- Forgetfulness	-- Diminished creativity	-- Negativity
-- Preoccupation		-- Denial

Social

-- Isolation	-- Quarreling	-- Lack of pleasure from experiences you usually enjoy
-- Uncomfortable being alone	-- Tension in relationships	
-- Sullenness	-- Dominating conversations	-- Blaming others
-- Defensiveness	-- Withdrawing from conversations	-- Nastiness

Occupational		
Caregiving work — Overwhelmed — Unprepared for tasks — Turned off by distasteful tasks — Difficulty making decisions/plans	— Feel no one understands — Carrying caregiving burdens alone — Conflict with other caregivers	
Employment/volunteer/home-based work — Worry about work during "off" hours — Coming to work late/leaving early — Less energy for, or interest in work — Being distracted; "there but not there"	— Lower than normal quality or productivity — Normal tasks are overwhelming — Absenteeism — Tardiness	
Spiritual		
— Doubt self-worth — Seeing life as meaningless — Hopelessness	— Loss of faith or ability to pray — Withdrawal from faith community	— Cynicism — Anger at God — Doubts about God — Asking, "Why me?"

©Partners on the Path. 2022. www.PartnersonthePath.com

Stressors Self-Care Activity #1: Interpreting My Score

A <u>short list</u> of checked items or one that has <u>no checks in several sections</u> suggests that you have few symptoms of stress. Most likely you are taking care of yourself and minimizing the impact that stress has on your life. It could be true that you have relatively little stress in your life. It is also possible that you are not aware of, or are not acknowledging signs that you are under stress.

A <u>long and diverse list</u> of stress symptoms is a sign that you may be at risk for developing stress-related illnesses, disruptions in your relationships with others or your ability to provide care. You may not be adequately attending to your needs or effectively managing your stress. It is also possible that you are experiencing a particularly intense time, and as a result your usual self-care practices may not be adequate to manage your stress.

If you have any question about your list, share it with a trusted friend, family member, counselor or clergy person; ask for their feedback. Also, situations change, so regularly reassess your stress symptoms to be aware of your need for self-care.

Stressors Self-Care Activity #2: Why am I so stressed?

Caregiving Stressors Checklist This checklist helps to name the caregiving tasks and challenges that are sources of your caregiver stress. Check all that apply to you. Also, this list can help you describe caregiving-related stress when seeking help from others.	
Caregiving Tasks	**Source of Stress**
1. **Physical Care:** I feed, bathe, dress, groom, or help with walking or getting to the bathroom. I do necessary medical/nursing tasks.	
2. **Personal Affairs**: I manage medicine, finances, legal, insurance, care coordination or transportation concerns.	
3. **Household Affairs**: I cook, clean, shop, launder clothes, do home repairs or help with relocation.	
4. **Emotional or Social Support**: I help with behavior, moods, socializing or making decisions.	
Caregiving Challenges	
1. **Unprecedented**: Since COVID, I am juggling an **increasing set of responsibilities** with **too little support** and often with **inadequate preparation or skill**.	
2. **Unprepared**: I am **responsible** for coordinating care or providing complex medical/nursing care, **yet have no medical training**.	
3. **Unpredictable**: I have **no control** over if, or when medical **emergencies and crises** will occur.	
4. **Unrealistic**: I manage **caregiving on top of my other responsibilities** to work, family and home. My "to-do" lists **have too many things I have to do**.	
5. **Unsupported**: I receive **inadequate help** from family or friends; from healthcare, insurance, legal or social service systems. It's **hard to get a break** from my responsibilities.	
6. **Upset**: I am grappling with **complicated emotions**, feelings of loss, anger, sadness, guilt, depression, or fear. I'm **unhappy with the "new normal"** that I have to live with.	
7. **Under-funded**: I may be **paying "out-of-pocket"** for caregiving supplies, services, or travel; **forging income**, or **spending my savings**. In general, caregiving is **hurting my finances**.	

©Partners on the Path. 2022. www.PartnersonthePath.com

Stressors Self-Care Activity #3: What kind of help do I need?

T-I-R-E-D Checklist Un-met needs are stressors that drain your energy. Use this list to identify your needs & to get the help you need.	
1. I need help with these *TASKS*:	√
Physical Care: Help to feed, bathe, dress, groom, or help to walk, get to bathroom; to perform medical/nursing tasks.	
Personal Affairs: Help to cook, clean, shop, launder clothes, run errands, do home repairs or help with relocation.	
Household Affairs: Help to manage medicine, finances, legal, insurance, care coordination or transportation.	
Emotional or Social Support: Help with behavior, moods, socializing or making decisions.	
2. I need this kind of *INFORMATION*:	√
Medical: Diagnosis/conditions, treatment options, professional referrals, health care organizations, medications, medical equipment	
Care Management: Community resources, national/state programs, professional care coordinators, medication management, online/technology resources, housing, senior driving advice	
Legal/Financial: Private and public insurance providers, eldercare attorneys, Veteran benefits	
3. I need this kind of break, or *RESPITE*:	√
Time out: Less than 30 minutes on an specific day/evening	
Mini-break: Several hours on a given day/evening	
Short getaway: Leave my loved one for a day or weekend	
Vacation: Leave my loved one for a week or more	

4. I need help in coping with *EMOTIONS related to these issues:*	√
Unprecedented: Since COVID, I am juggling an **increasing set of responsibilities** with **too little support** and often with **inadequate preparation or skill**.	
Unprepared: I am **responsible** for managing care or providing complex medical/nursing care, **yet have no medical training**.	
Unpredictable: I have **no control** over if or when medical **emergencies and crises** will occur.	
Unrealistic: I manage **caregiving on top of other responsibilities** to work, family and home. My **"to-do" lists is too much!**	
Unsupported: I receive **inadequate help** from family, friends, health care, insurance or legal systems. It's **hard to get a break** from my responsibilities.	
Upset: I am grappling with **complicated emotions**, feelings of loss, anger, sadness, guilt, depression, or fear. I'm unhappy with the **"new normal"** that I'm forced to accept.	
Under-funded: Paying **"out-of-pocket" for caregiving expenses** (supplies, services, or travel) is **hurting my finances**.	
5. I need help making *DECISIONS* like these:	√
Workplace issues-How to handle: Overload of work & caregiving responsibilities; conflict-culture isn't caregiver-friendly; need change & need income	
Family or personal issues-How to handle: Unbalanced family involvement; conflict; different caregiving priorities; loneliness; need for self-care	
Health care or medical treatment issues-How to handle: Problems with physical or mental health; cost/time barriers to staying healthy	
Legal or financial issues-How to handle: Costs of caregiving supplies, services or travel; loss of income/savings; power-of-attorney	

©Partners on the Path. 2022. www.PartnersonthePath.com

Helpful Resources

Abramson, Alexis. *The Caregiver's Survival Handbook*. Perigee, 2011.

Caring for the Caregiver: Consider the Facts https://www.youtube.com/watch?v=tz1KGUQvYNU&t=86s and

Caregiver Concerns: How do I recognize the need for self-care? https://www.youtube.com/watch?v=SFUlv6igwJI Two YouTube videos of the author describing caregiver stress and the need for self-care.

Davis, Martha et.al. *The Relaxation & Stress Reduction Workbook. 7ᵗʰ edition*. New Harbinger. 2019.

Help Guide: https://www.helpguide.org/ offers trustworthy, ad-free information and resources for dealing with challenging mental health and wellness issues. Content focuses on mental and emotional health, family and relationships, wellness, and aging. They also offer exclusive content from Harvard Health Publishing, the consumer health publishing division of Harvard Medical School.

Jacobs, Barry. *The Emotional Survival Guide for Caregivers.* The Guilford Press, 2006.

Loverde, Joy. *The Complete Eldercare Planner.* Harmony. 2009.

"One critical step to easing the stress—and guilt—of caregiving is to admit that you can't do it alone and to seek help. Many caregivers rely on a combination of family and paid help."
Alexis Abramson
Author of The Caregiver's Survival Handbook

"The greatest weapon against stress is our ability to choose one thought over the other."
William James
American philosopher and psychologist

"One of the best pieces of advice I ever got was from a horse master. He told me to go slow to go fast. I think that applies to everything in life. We live as though there aren't enough hours in the day but if we do each thing calmly and carefully we will get it done quicker and with much less stress."
Viggo Mortensen
American actor and musician

CHAPTER 4

The Toll: Consequences of Caregiver Stress

Jane's Story: Support Group

You want me to do what!? Attend a support group? Yeah, right! I could fit that in after my ten-hour day at work, just before I stop to buy the Depends for my mom, on the way to pick up the kids from practice and go home to make dinner. Or, maybe after dinner, when the dishes are cleared and I've finally managed to get the kids off the computer and phone and on to their homework. Or, perhaps between doing loads of laundry and calling my brothers to remind them that Mom is doing OK, but would really like to see them. You want me to take time for myself!? I don't see how I could possibly do one more thing, even if it is something good for me. It would just stress me out more to try to make the arrangements.

Sometimes words like these form in my mind, or actually come out of my mouth when others suggest I take a break from the rigors of caregiving. I dismiss others' suggestions for self-care. Why do I do this? Am I in such a rut that I can't see even just a few ways to reprioritize, reorganize, or reschedule parts of life so I can grab some time for me? Am I feeling so unworthy that I believe everyone else's needs really are more important than mine? Am I feeling so guilty to be healthy when Mom is suffering, that I won't allow myself to stop; so blind to the consequences of living an over-extended life that I can't see the real possibility of becoming sick from too much stress?

Whatever the reasons, taking some kind of self-care action now is more important than understanding why I haven't until now. What I need is some respite, a break that will help me relax and regain some energy. Maybe finding time to go out to a support group is beyond what I can do today. But I know there are lots of other things that can relieve my stress and give me strength for the journey ahead. I just need to do some of them.

How are you caring for yourself?

I went through a period during my caregiving years when I was always sick, nothing really serious but mostly annoying and inconvenient. A series of sinus infections plagued me for years. On the plane ride home from one trip to see my Mom, I contracted a nasty virus which was not diagnosed for three months, and which kept me sick and tired for another three months. I was depressed and my immune system was shot. I spent more days in bed that winter than I had since infancy! Feeling lucky that it was nothing more serious, I realized that caregiving had silently stolen my vitality. How are you? Are you experiencing any signs of strain? What have you done for yourself lately? If you need to take better care of yourself, here are a few ideas that might be useful.

Self-Care Recommendations

What is self-care and why is it important?

Relief from the stress of caregiving starts with recognizing the importance of self-care and practicing it regularly. *What is self-care?* Self-care is being concerned about yourself, as well as others; looking out for your own welfare, making sure that your needs are met, not only those of others. Self-care is that collection of choices you make and behaviors you practice that make you feel good, solve your problems and ultimately, relieve your stress.

Managing stress by practicing *self-care is important* because it protects your health, helps you cope when the things that cause stress are beyond your control, and helps you maintain the balance you require to care in a loving and effective way. To see how caregiving is impacting your well-being, complete the **Burden Scale for Family Caregivers** found in the this chapter's *Self-Care Activity #1: Is my health "at risk" because of caregiving?*

How can I practice self-care? Use the six steps listed below.

1: Name your symptoms and sources of stress

All successful self-care starts here. To help name your symptoms and sources of caregiver stress, refer back to two checklists found in Chapter 3:

- *Stressors Self-Care Activity #1: What are my symptoms of caregiver stress?*
- *Stressors Self-Care Activity #2: Why am I so stressed?*

2: Adjust your attitude

You can control the wear and tear of distress you experience by adjusting your attitude in the following ways:

- **Using positive self-talk**: Silently or aloud affirm your strength and ability to cope. Say to yourself, "I can do this!"

- **Challenging negative beliefs**: Question negative assumptions. Consider possible positive outcomes. Ask yourself, "What is the worst that could happen? What is the best that could happen? What is most likely to happen?"

- **Relabeling**: Think and talk about stress from a positive, not a negative perspective. Replace, "This is an awful problem." Instead think, "This is a challenge or opportunity."

3: Decide on a course of action

Ask yourself: *Is there anything I can do to change or eliminate the stressors in my life?* A yes or no answer leads to different approaches to self-care. Here are two examples.

Imagine your stressor is a disagreement with others over division of caregiving tasks. You are tired, have other pressing responsibilities and need some help. In this case your answer to the question would be, "Yes. If I take some action the stressor could be relieved, or will completely go away. My friends or family may help me if I ask them." *When you control or can influence stressors, the best course of action is assertiveness and problem solving.* This approach will yield relief and may even eliminate your stressors. Be sure to use a positive approach when solving problems.

In a second scenario, the stressor is your loved one's Alzheimer's disease, the progression of their illness and the suffering that goes with it. Here your answer to the question would be, "No. No matter what I do the diagnosis won't change or go away. I need to find some way to live with this." *When you have no control or influence over your stressor, the best course of action is using healthy self-care practices.* Problem solving or assertiveness won't have an effect. Self-care helps you retain energy and feel better when stressors are beyond your control.

One caution: Take care that you don't reply "no" to the question of your ability to change or eliminate stress when, with courage, you could answer "yes." Check your perceptions with a reliable person.

4: Use healthy self-care practices daily, and at times when you lack control

Loss of control is very stressful. *When there is nothing to be done, the thing you CAN do is care for yourself.* Don't wait until you have already worn down; *make self-care a priority in your daily routine.* Choose things that are self-soothing–whatever helps you calm down, have fun, relax, enjoy or feel pampered. When called for, choose things that involve self-discipline; although less pleasurable, in the long run, disciplined self-care practices lead to a greater sense of well-being. You will find a checklist of healthy self-care practices in the Activities section of this chapter: *The Toll Activity #2: What healthy self-care practices do I currently use?*

5: Avoid stress-numbing behaviors

Stress-numbing behaviors include: complaining and blaming; drugs and drinking; over eating and consuming junk food; buying sprees; smoking; sleeping to avoid stress; burying yourself in television, video games, the computer or other distractions; or avoiding action on problem-solving. *These behaviors numb the distress of being a caregiver, but do nothing to help body, mind or spirit cope in a healthy way.* By promoting a sense of release or relaxation, they give the illusion of self-care, but if overused, or used in place of problem-solving action, can actually create more stress than they relieve.

What stress-numbing behaviors do you use? How much do you rely on them to dull the pain or discomfort in your life? Make sure that these are not big parts of your approach to self-care. If you are too reliant on any of these practices, look for alternatives that are healthier and more effective.

6: Use problem-solving skills when you have control

When some action on your part can ease or eliminate your stress, take problem-solving action by using this four-step process.

Step 1: Figure out what your problem is:

Name the challenge, opportunity, difficulty, or situation that needs improvement. If emotions or confusion makes this difficult, ask those you respect and trust for help. Organize your facts:

- WHO contributed to this problem? WHO was affected?
- WHAT happened to create this problem: violated expectations or promises, bad behavior, something else?
- WHEN did this happen?
- WHERE did this happen?
- HOW do you and others feel in response to this problem?
- WHY is this important?

Step 2: Develop a problem-solving plan.

- *Consider options.* Ask: What can be done to resolve this problem? Brainstorm to develop possible solutions; the more options you create, the more likely you will identify an effective solution.

- *State desired outcomes.* Ask: What do I want to achieve? What are short and long-term goals? What rewards will I get if this problem is solved?

- *Write an action plan.* Create a three-column chart with these headings and fill in the details.

    1. WHAT: Name each step and the tasks for accomplishing it. Think about what difficulties might arise and how you could handle them.

2. WHO: Name the person(s) who will be responsible for doing each step of the plan.

3. WHEN: Identify deadlines for completing each task.

Step 3: Carry-out your plan.

Take action and check for progress. Tracking progress is critical; it will motivate you to follow through on the plan. Remind those involved of deadlines for each step and for the whole plan, the desired outcomes, and rewards for success.

Step 4: Evaluate your plan.

- Did we solve the problem? Did we achieve our goal?
- Did we change the situation? What worked? What didn't work?
- Are we listening to all feedback, both positive and critical? What have we learned?
- Does anything more need to be done?

Activities for Caregivers

The Toll Self-Care Activity #1: Is my health "at risk" because of caregiving?

Burden Scale for Family Caregivers-Short version (BSFC-s) Consider your present caregiving situation, the type of assistance you provide and responsibilities associated with the condition or illness of you family member or friend. **For each item, select the number that best describes your present situation. Please answer all ten items!**				
	Strongly Agree	**Agree**	**Disagree**	**Strongly Disagree**
1. My life satisfaction has suffered because of the care I give.	3	2	1	0
2. I often feel physically exhausted.	3	2	1	0
3. From time to time I wish I could "run away" from the situation I am in.	3	2	1	0
4. Sometimes I don't really feel like "myself" as I did before.	3	2	1	0
5. Since I have been a caregiver my financial situation has been negatively affected.	3	2	1	0
6. My health is affected by the care situation.	3	2	1	0

7. The care I give takes a lot of my own strength.	**3**	**2**	**1**	**0**
8. I feel torn between the demands of my environment (such as family or work) and the demands of the care I give.	**3**	**2**	**1**	**0**
9. I am worried about my future because of the care I give.	**3**	**2**	**1**	**0**
10. My relationships with other family members, relatives, friends and acquaintances are suffering as a result of the care I give.	**3**	**2**	**1**	**0**
Scoring: Add-up the numbers you circled. **To interpret your score, see the Scoring Guide.**	**My score is:** _____			
Source: Graessel Berth *et al. BMC Geriatrics* 2014, 14:23 (open access) **www. caregiver-burden.eu**				

The Toll Activity #1: Burden Scale for Family Caregivers (BSFC-s) Scoring Guide

<u>Scoring Guide</u>: Use this guide to understand your scores, and to consider ways to protect your health.

<u>A total score of 0-5</u> indicates that you are experiencing a few physical complaints, or none at all. Based on this score, your level of physical problems is in line with the general population. Your caregiving situation has not increased your risk for impaired health.

<u>A total score of 6-14</u> indicates that you are experiencing a somewhat or moderately higher level of physical complaints. As a result of your caregiving situation, you are at increased risk for impaired health.

<u>A total score of 15-30</u> indicates that you are experiencing a severe to very severe rise in physical complaints. Your caregiving situation has significantly increased your risk for impaired health.

<u>Your scores can change over time</u>; check yourself again in the future to remain aware of your situation.

©Elmar Graessel, Hendrik Berth, Thomas Lichte, Hannes Grau, Anna Pendergrass, Cintia Malnis, Uta Graf, Sabine Engel. 2017. Used with permission.

The Toll Activity #2: What healthy self-care practices do I currently use?

Self-Care Checklist		
Check the self-care practices you use. In the future, aim for diversity and frequency in self-care; it's best for your health!		
Physical		
-- Exercise regularly -- Rest during the day -- Sleep 7-8 hours at night -- Eat a balanced diet -- Limit "junk food" -- Drink eight glasses of water daily	-- Maintain weight in desired range -- Limit alcohol consumption -- Do not smoke -- Use medications as prescribed __ Visit physician for check-ups __ Practice yoga	-- Practice the relaxation response -- Groom yourself – manicure, facial, haircut, shave, etc. -- Get a massage __ Receive chiropractic care __ Practice Reiki __ Engage in outdoor activities
Emotional		
-- Allow yourself to feel emotions -- Appropriately & respectfully express emotions -- Work off anger with physical exercise -- Say "no" when you want or need to -- Ask directly for what you want	-- Cry -- Laugh -- Resolve conflicts -- Nurture yourself -- Don't take things too seriously	
Mental		
-- Ask questions -- Accept ambiguity -- Read -- Take risks __ Practice guided imagery	-- Daydream -- Learn something new -- Consider different viewpoints -- Read self-help books __ Use visualization or affirmation	-- Relabel unpleasant situations -- Develop plans -- Think optimistically -- Use helpful web-based resources __ Take responsibility for yourself/your life
Social		
-- Develop and use support systems -- Talk with friends and family -- Take time off -- Go on vacation -- Rehabilitate or end unsatisfactory relationships -- Limit TV viewing -- Engage in a creative pastime or hobby	-- Read humorous books/watch humorous shows -- Socialize with others -- Enjoy intimacy or sex -- Play -- Spend time alone -- Treat yourself to something enjoyable: new clothes, CD's, magazine, etc. -- Engage in volunteer activities	

Spiritual		
–– Pray or meditate –– Commune with nature –– "Let go" of unsolvable problems	–– Attend worship services –– Read inspirational prose or poetry –– Appreciate the beauty of art or music	–– Take one day at a time –– Clarify your values and beliefs –– Acknowledge your self-worth

Occupational: Employment and/or Caregiving Work	
–– Learn new skills –– Pace yourself –– Balance involvement and detachment –– Seek respite-daily, periodic, short term, or vacations –– Get organized –– Take breaks –– Do your best and let go of the rest	–– Share responsibilities with others –– Let others sometimes do a stressful/difficult task –– Beautify your environment –– Acknowledge the good you do –– Leave work at work –– Develop good relationships with co-workers –– Open yourself to change __ Use Employee Assistance Program/your employer's helpful resources

Problem Solving Action	
__ Effectively manage time __ Assertively communicate with others __ Negotiate with others for desired outcomes __ Constructively resolve conflict __ Create a comfortable home	__ Learn new information or life skills __ Change dysfunctional/self-defeating behaviors __ Clarify or resolve misunderstandings __ Budget and wisely manage finances __ Keep possessions in good working order

©Partners on the Path. 2020. www.PartnersonthePath.com

The Toll Activity #3: Problem-Solving Process

<u>**Self-Care: Guided Self-Reflection**</u>
Directions: Refer back to the four-step problem-solving process, described in this chapter. Use these steps to help you outline how you will solve a specific caregiving problem you are currently facing. Seek ideas from others to help you choose your best course of action.

Step 1: MY PROBLEM Name one caregiving problem.

Step 2: MY ACTION PLAN Develop a plan for solving your problem: GOAL? WHAT? WHO? WHEN?
Use another paper if you need more space.

GOAL: The outcome I am seeking.

WHAT: Name each step or task for accomplishing the outcomes I desire.	**WHO:** Person(s) responsible for this step or task	**WHEN:** Identify deadlines for completing each step or task.

Step 3: CARRY-OUT YOUR PLAN Take action and track progress toward you goal.
HOW will you monitor progress? How will you assure that deadlines are met? How will you reward success?

Step 4: EVALUATE YOUR PLAN Answer the following questions:

    1. Did we solve the problem?

    2. Did we achieve our goal?

    3. Did we change the situation?

    4. Are we listening to all feedback, both positive and critical?

    5. Does anything more need to be done?

    6. What have we learned from this situation?

    7. What worked? What didn't work?

The Toll Activity #4: Guided Self-Reflection

Self-Care: Guided Self-Reflection
Directions: Think about your current self-care practices. Respond to the following questions to help clarify which ones are helpful and healthy and which are not. Promise to do something good for yourself today!

1.	My Attitude and Thoughts

Name It
- If I adjust my attitude, would that help relieve some of my stress?
- What are the negative thoughts I should let go and what positive thoughts should replace them?

2.	Stress Numbing Behaviors

Name It
- What stress-numbing behaviors do I turn to for relief?
- Am I overly reliant on these?
- What healthier practices could replace some of my current stress-numbing behaviors?

3.	Healthy Self-Care Practices

Name It
- What healthy self-care practices have already helped me handle stressors that are beyond my control?
- Are there any new behaviors or practices that I could add: things that are soothing, fun, energizing, relaxing, or feel like a treat?
- **What one or two things will I do to care for myself today?**

Helpful Resources

Berman, Claire. ***Caring for Yourself while Caring for Your Aging Parents***. 3rd Edition. Holt Paperbacks. 2005.

Caring for the Caregiver: Care for yourself as you care for others https://youtu.be/JIwMg79w598 YouTube video from the author describing the importance of self-care.

Caregiver Questions is a You-Tube video series from the author that answers caregivers' questions about self-care.

1. ***What is self-care?*** https://www.youtube.com/watch?v=X2v1PNuE_GM&t=78s

2. ***Why is self-care important?*** https://www.youtube.com/watch?v=HUi5MATqQY8

3. ***What makes self-care difficult?*** https://www.youtube.com/watch?v=YW7y3JzRwaY

4. ***How do I find the time for self-care?*** https://vimeo.com/189002148

5. ***Do little things really make a difference?*** https://www.youtube.com/watch?v=y76wqg4rMow

Jacobs, Barry and Mayer, Julia. ***Meditations for Caregivers: Practical, Emotional, and Spiritual Support for You and Your Family***. Da Capo Press. 2016.

Lotsa Helping Hands: https://lotsahelpinghands.com/ offers a secure site that you can use to organize family, friends, neighbors, and colleagues during times of need. It allows you to easily coordinate activities and manage volunteers with an intuitive group calendar. You can also communicate and share information using announcements, messages boards and photos. A Lotsa App can be downloaded from the <u>App Store</u> or <u>Google Play Store</u>.

Shaw, Zoe. ***A Year of Self-Care: Daily Practices and Inspiration for Caring for Yourself (A Year of Daily Reflections).*** Rockridge Press. 2021.

....

"To keep the body in good health is a duty…otherwise we will not be able to keep our mind strong and clear."
Buddah
Philosopher, teacher, founder of Buddhism

"Forget the times of your distress, but never forget what they taught you."
Robert C. Gallagher
Author

"To give good care to others, we first must take care of ourselves. We can become handicapped as caregivers not because we lack knowledge about durable powers of attorney or long-term care insurance…but because we exclude ourselves from the care equation."
Beth Witrogen McLeod
Speaker and author of *Caregiving: The Spiritual Journey of Love, Loss and Renewal*

....

CHAPTER 5

3 Things Every Caregiver Needs

Caring for others is often deeply meaningful but it's never easy. It can take a toll on body and mind, heart and soul, on finances, family and work life. Lessons I've learned over the years are the core of what I'll share in this book. One of the most important facts about caregivers is this:

All caregivers need 3 things.

1. **Practical, Problem-Solving Resources:** Caregivers need information, skills, and resources to do the work of caregiving.

   - Links, references or referrals
   - Answers to questions and guidance on solving problems;
   - Help with specific tasks or challenges
   - New skills required for effective functioning as a caregiver or in other roles
   - People who will provide hands-on help

2. **Positive Personal Energy:** Caregivers need physical and emotional resilience to meet challenges they encounter on their journey. Necessary strength and stamina are developed by consciously choosing thoughts, attitudes, and actions that protect and restore vitality.

- Meeting adversity with optimism.
- Protecting good health.
- Cultivating social support and spiritual practices.
- Avoiding stress-numbing behaviors.
- Prioritizing and regularly practicing healthy self-care.

3. **Partners in Providing Care:** Caregivers need to connect with care partners who will help them: do the work of caregiving; persevere throughout their caregiving journey; and know that they are not alone.

   - Cultivating a supportive community which includes family, friends and fellow-caregivers; professionals, work colleagues, neighbors, and faith-community members.
   - Actively seeking those who are compassionate, effective and reliable
   - Connecting with those who respond when asked for assistance
   - Avoiding toxic, negative, or overly critical.

What about you?

To stay healthy and capable of meeting caregiving challenges, be sure to take care of your needs, not just those of others.

Activities for Caregivers

Caregiver Needs Activity #1: Recognizing My Needs

<u>**My Unmet Needs: Guided Self-Reflection**</u> **<u>Directions</u>:** Think about what you need to handle caregiving tasks and challenges. Awareness of your needs is an important first step in getting the help you need.
1.   **<u>Practical Problem-Solving Resources</u>**: Information, links or referrals that would help me handle my caregiving tasks and challenges. Skills I need but don't have, or am uncomfortable doing. Times when I need hands-on help.

<u>**Name It**</u>
  • What practical problem-solving resources do you need to assist you with caregiving responsibilities?
  • How does lacking these resources impact you?

2.   **<u>Positive Personal Energy</u>**: Actions would nurture me and refresh my energy. Thoughts and attitudes that would strengthen me to meet adversity with optimism and effectively handle caregiving-related challenges.

<u>**Name It**</u>
  • Where or when is your energy either diminished or negative?
  • What causes this to occur?
  • How does this diminished or negative energy impact you?

3.	**Partners on the Path:** Names of family, friends & fellow-caregivers; work colleagues, neighbors, faith-community members and professionals who could help. Where I could go for support & assurance that I'm not alone.

Name It
- In what aspects of caregiving do your feel unsupported or alone?
- What kind of support do you need? To whom or where could you turn for help?
- How does the lack of effective care partners impact you?

©Partners on the Path. 2022. www.PartnersonthePath.com

Caregiver Needs Activity #2: Meeting My Needs

<table>
<tr><td>
<u>**Meeting My Needs: Action Plan**</u>
Directions: After naming what you need to handle caregiving tasks and challenges, identify at least one thing you'll do to care for yourself as you care for others.
<u>To preserve your capacity to care: Admit, permit & commit to following your self-care action plan.</u>
</td></tr>
<tr><td>
1.   <u>**Practical Problem-Solving Resources**</u>: Information, links or referrals that will help me handle my caregiving tasks and challenges. New skills I'll develop. People I'll ask for hands-on help.
</td></tr>
<tr><td>
•   <u>**Name It:**</u> What practical problem-solving resources do you need to assist you with caregiving responsibilities?
</td></tr>
<tr><td>
•   <u>**Get It:**</u> Who will you ask? What will you ask for? Where will you seek-out problem-solving resources?
</td></tr>
<tr><td>
2.   <u>**Positive Personal Energy**</u>: Actions I'll take that will nurture me and refresh my energy. Thoughts and attitudes I'll use to help me meet adversity with optimism and resilience.
</td></tr>
<tr><td>
•   <u>**Name It:**</u> Where or when is your energy either diminished or negative? What causes this to occur?
</td></tr>
<tr><td>
•   <u>**Get It:**</u> What thoughts, attitudes or actions have restored your energy in the past? What will you do to boost your positive energy?
</td></tr>
</table>

3. **Partners on the Path:** Names of family, friends and fellow-caregivers; work colleagues, neighbors, faith-community members and professionals who I'll reach-out to for help, support & assurance that I'm not alone.

- **Name It:** In what aspects of caregiving do your feel unsupported or alone? What kind of support do you need?

- **Get It:** Who will you ask for assistance or support? What will you say to make the request and to explain your need for caregiving partners?

Helpful Resources

AARP's Caregiver Resource Center: https://www.aarp.org/caregiving/ offers a robust array of information, tools and guides. Use the dropdown menus to search for guidance: 1-Basics; 2-Care at Home; 3-Medical; 4-Financial & Legal; 5- Caregiver Life Balance; 6-Community; 7-Local Resources & Solutions; 8-Stories.

Caregiver Concerns: I feel so exhausted! https://www.youtube.com/ watch?v=j1zeeWfrRoo&t=2s a YouTube video from the author about strategies for addressing energy depletion.

Green, Eboni. ***Caregiving in the New Millennium: 3rd Edition.*** 2021. Green Publishing.

You'll be Okay: https://vimeo.com/18023045 YouTube video in which the author highlights the value of small acts of self-care.

....

"Don't neglect your own needs. Remember those airplane safety movies that instruct you to put your own oxygen mask on first, before assisting a child or someone who needs help? The logic is that you won't be much help to anyone if you are disoriented or passed out yourself."
Sasha Carr and Sandra Choron
Co-authors of *The Caregiver's Essential Handbook*

"Everybody needs beauty as well as bread, places to play in and pray in, where nature may heal and give strength to body and soul."
John Muir
Scottish-American naturalist and "Father of the National Parks"

....

CHAPTER 6

Self-Care: Necessary for Well-Being

Simply put, *self-care is anything healthy that you do to protect or promote your own well-being.* Self-care is a **holistic** approach to self-nurture, feeding any and all aspects of your human life: physical, emotional, mental, social, occupational or spiritual. *Feeding any part of you energizes all of you.*

Self-care is any **healthy** activity that fosters well-being. By nurturing yourself, you can stay healthy and functional as a caregiver, and in others aspects of your life. Self-care avoids stress-numbing behaviors like smoking, eating junk food, or excess eating and drinking. *In the absence of self-care, you are vulnerable to stress related illnesses.*

Self-care is **personalized & restorative**: doing specific things that address your particular needs; taking specific actions that relieve your stress and that replenish your positive energy. Self-care involves putting your needs on the "to-do" list along with those of others. It is following the airplane advice to "put your oxygen mask on before trying to help others" because, *as a caregiver, you can't help if you can't function.*

Self-care is not something that's simply "nice-to-do," something that can be ignored without consequences. It is **necessary** if you want to remain healthy and continue providing care. Like other caregivers who are overloaded with responsibilities, you may ask, "How can I FIND the time for self-care?" If health and well-being are important, it helps to change the question. Instead, ask, *"How do I MAKE time for self-care?"* *The answer is to admit, permit and commit to practicing healthy self-care.*

Admit, Permit & Commit to Healthy Self-Care

1. **Admit to needing self-care.** *You are a human being, not a "caregiving machine"* that plugs into an electrical socket for energy. You aren't the Energizer Bunny with endless energy, powered by batteries. No, your human energy is natural and comes from within. It ebbs and flows; when energy is spent it must be replenished. *Self-care practices restore energy for caregiving.*

   Juggling and struggling with caregiving takes a toll. Overlooking the cost of over-functioning leaves you vulnerable to stress related illness. So stop minimizing or denying how the challenges of caregiving impact your well-being. Take the first step and admit to your need for self-care.

2. **Permit yourself to act on your own behalf.** Think about what keeps you from self-care. Is it guilt about taking time for yourself when others have so much need? Questioning the importance of self-care? Doubting that small acts of self-care add up to much of anything? Research shows that self-care positively impacts physical and mental health. *Self-care isn't selfish; it's a valuable health promotion activity.*

   Reframe your thoughts about self-care; view it as a healthy habit, like daily dental care. Brushing with a good toothpaste and flossing regularly is a daily routine that takes little time or much thought. But done every day for years, these small acts add up to significant dental health. Self-care is just like this; little healthy acts, every day, add up to a healthier you. So think of self-care as OK to do, as wise, as a necessity for a healthy life.

3. **Commit to daily action.** Refute doubts about the effect of self-care. Picture putting one or two pennies into a glass jar every day. As weeks turn into months and an entire year passes, a

couple of pennies add up to a jar that is overflowing. Small, daily acts of self-care are just like those coins; your daily deposits fill you up.

Put yourself on your "to-do" list. Promise to care for yourself, just as you care for others. Do whatever relieves stress and brings you joy: stretching, deep breathing, appreciating nature or art, talking with a friend, praying, petting your dog or cat, exercising, playing with a child, playing an instrument, singing or dancing, holding someone's hand, offering a compliment, napping, figuring out how to solve a problem, or asking for help. The options are endless.

Plan & follow-through on your commitment to self-care; put those pennies in the jar each day and watch them accumulate. As with any healthy habit, the more you do it, the easier it becomes. *Practiced daily, self-care actions that are as seemingly insignificant as a penny soon add up to a healthier you.* When self-care becomes your habit, you'll FIND the time because you've MADE time for self-care. Watch the author's YouTube video on finding the time by making the time for self-care: https://www.youtube.com/watch?v=WvVD7blt29A

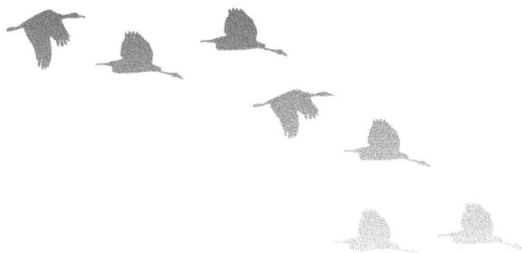

CHAPTER 7

Self-Care: Replenish Your Energy

Jane's Story: What am I made of?

I feel really worn down and blue today. Caring for Mom and Dad is both a joy and a burden; deeply inspiring and repetitiously boring. It fills my heart and drains the last drop of energy I have; makes me proud of what I can do for my parents, yet guilty that I'm mad about having to do it. For twenty years I've cared for different people in my family. Right now I'm at a low point; caregiving is an arduous journey. My sister, Wendy, just sent me an email, one of those stories that circulate on the web, author unknown. Somehow, this anonymous little tale really speaks to me, as if Wendy wrote it just for me. The story from the web is titled *Carrots, Eggs or Coffee?* It goes like this:

> A young woman went to talk with her mother and share how hard her life was. She didn't know how she was going to make it and wanted to give up; she was tired of struggling. It seemed as if when one problem was solved, a new one arose.
>
> The girl's mother took her to the kitchen. She filled three pots with water, and put them on the stove to boil. In the first, she placed carrots. In the second she placed eggs, and in the last pot, she placed ground coffee beans. The mother let them sit and boil without saying a word.

After twenty minutes, Mom turned off the burners, fished out the carrots and placed them in a bowl, removed the eggs from the second pot, and poured the steaming, aromatic coffee into a large mug. Turning to her daughter, the mother asked, "What do you see?" "Carrots, eggs and coffee," the young woman replied, wondering where this was going. The mother asked her daughter to feel the carrots, peel the hard-boiled egg, and sip the cup of coffee.

Finally revealing the meaning of this odd exercise, the mother explained that each of these objects had faced the same "adversity," boiling water, but each had reacted differently. The carrot went in strong, firm, and unrelenting. However, after being subjected to boiling water, it softened and became weak. The egg had been fragile, with a thin outer shell protecting its fluid interior. Like the carrots, the egg was changed by the boiling water. Its soft interior became hardened.

The mother pointed out that the coffee was unique; it alone had changed the water in which it had been boiled and turned it into something quite wonderful. Then she asked her troubled daughter, "Which one are you? In the face of adversity will you wilt and go soft, like the carrot? Will your fluid spirit harden, or, like the coffee beans, will you release the potential within you and turn the boiling waters of your life into something you savor?"

What are you made of?

Faced with adversity, what are you like: the carrot, eggs or coffee? Do you have the energy, judgment and grace to persevere with caregiving? By centering yourself, you can tap into the wisdom and calm at your core and be like the coffee. Here are some ideas about how to do that.

Self-Care Recommendations

I am so overloaded! Why should I take the time for centering?

Would you like to handle caregiving with internal peace, balance and focused energy? These characteristics are always present deep inside you, no matter what intense emotions or anxious worries are churning within, no matter how tumultuous external events may be. They are always available if you are willing to reach for them, and if you develop the ability to connect with them through the practice of centering.

What can I do to feel more centered in my caregiving?

1. **Recognize the source of your energy.** As a human being, your life energy flows from living in harmony and balance, staying in tune with three factors:

   - **Universal principles**: Do unto others as you would have them do unto you. To everything there is a season. Honor your father and your mother. As you sow, so shall you reap. No man is an island. *Violating universal principles like these creates disharmony and drains you.* Follow universal principles.

   - **Your human nature**: You are physical, emotional, mental, social, and spiritual. Your personal energy flows when these five elements balance with the sixth element, the work that you do. *Caring for all parts of yourself fills you with positive energy and helps you retain balance.* Nurture all parts of yourself.

   - **Your unique identity**: What distinguishes you from others? You have strengths and weaknesses; personal skills, qualities and a ways of doing things; values and principles that help you handle life challenges. *Your life is richer and more satisfying when you know and respect your uniqueness.* Be true to yourself.

2. **Understand how your energy flows.** You are human, not a machine. You are alive, operating on natural, not mechanical energy. You don't

plug yourself in each morning and operate continuously like your computer or radio. You have cycles, with ups and downs. Like hours in a day or seasons in a year, your energy ebbs and flows. Your energy is affected by your environment. What goes on around you feeds or drains you, unlike machines that operate the same, whether the room is bright or dark. *Accept and work with the natural flow of your energy* so you can continue helping the ones you love.

3. **Balance involvement and detachment.** Balancing is the dynamic process of adapting to changing or competing demands. It involves *consciously choosing what you will and won't do, based on what you can and can't handle.* Balancing helps you avoid both dysfunctional over-involvement and distant disengagement from your caregiving role. Neither is healthy for you, your care receiver or other caregivers working with you. Make readjustments to recover balance if you have become over-involved or disengaged from your caregiving role. Be realistic about your limits; live within them to remain in balance. Say "No" to activities that draw you beyond what is reasonable for you to manage. Find alternative ways to deal with what you're unable to handle.

4. **Acknowledge your pain.** Bound together by the ties of family or friendship, you are affected by your loved one's condition. Though separate bodies, you are connected in your hearts and souls. Both of you grapple with intangible yet real heartaches that can take the form of distressing thoughts, feelings or physical symptoms. Borne alone, heartache slowly but inevitably erodes energy, health and peace of mind. Acknowledging your pain and sharing it with a trusted friend, counselor, member of your family or the clergy can help you. *Open up and talk about your feelings.*

5. **Conserve your energy**. *Your energy is finite.* Conserving your energy involves wise choices that must be made daily. Not always easy to make, they involve saying "no" to habits that waste time and energy.

- *Define important.* Save energy for what is important, not just what seems urgent.

- *Eliminate the unimportant.* You can't do everything. Trim away non-essentials.

- *Sequence activities.* Work on large projects step-by-step. Postpone what could be done later.

- *Simplify your life.* Pare down what is complex or elaborate. Say "no" to overloading your schedule.

- *Avoid toxicity.* Stay away from people or situations that drag you down, erode your confidence or threaten your safety.

- *Let go of what you do not control.* However hard you try, well you plan, or carefully you communicate, you control very little of the total caregiving situation.

6. Replenish your energy. *Use these four simple, but powerful techniques to center yourself and reenergize.*

- **Breathe like a baby.** Deep breathing lowers your heart rate, anxiety and muscle tension. It is the easiest way to elicit the relaxation response. In moments of high stress, pay attention to your breathing; breathe slowly and deeply from your abdomen. For the on-going stress of caregiving, make it a practice to breathe slowly and deeply for at least three minutes every day.

- **Clear your mind.** Worry, uncertainty and anxiety are frequent partners on the path of caregiving. They can escalate into catastrophic thinking that makes life miserable, wastes time, and interferes with effective problem-solving. Methods for clearing your mind include silence, prayer, meditation, journal writing, art, solitude, and communing with nature.

- **Pursue your dreams**. Caring for your loved one isn't an either/or proposition; either your loved one's needs are met or yours are. It is more a question of finding ways to take good care of both your loved one and yourself. Pursuing what gives you joy and satisfaction, if only on a small scale, keeps the spark in your life and supplies energy to continue caring, however long and hard the journey. Take care not to put your dreams on hold.

- **Borrow from others**. The surest way to protect your health and restore depleted energy is to borrow some from your network. Reach out to anyone who could help: friends, family, people in your faith community or neighborhood, volunteers from community organizations, professional contacts, and people you could hire. Ask for help with caregiving work, or managing aspects of your own affairs that are hard to get to because of caregiving responsibilities.

One last thought…

Centering yourself as a caregiver is like preparing to climb a tall mountain. You cannot reach the summit without strength and stamina. Building–up your capacity to meet the challenges of an arduous journey is hard work. It takes commitment, wisdom, practice and patience. Persevering until you reach your goal demands regular refueling and periods of rest along the way. *In caregiving, your ability to meet the challenge starts with an awareness of your needs and a commitment to caring in a balanced way. Start small, take your time, pace yourself and refuel regularly.* With consistent focus on centering, you will develop the physical, emotional, and spiritual capacity to care…however long or demanding your journey.

Activities for Caregivers

Replenish Your Energy Activity #1: How balanced is my involvement in caregiving?

<u>Caregiving Balance Checklist</u>
Balancing helps you adapt to life's changing or competing demands. It helps you stay resilient and healthy. It helps you avoid both *unhealthy over-involvement* and *harmful disengagement* from your caregiver role. Neither is healthy for you, your care receiver or other caregivers working with you to provide care.

Directions: Read through the seven descriptions below. Check the item that best describes your current approach to caregiving.

____	**1. Detached:** You demonstrate no concern for the physical or emotional well-being of your loved one. You are disinterested and/or uninvolved in providing any type of care.
____	**2. Distant:** With prompting from others, you experience some concern about the well-being of your loved one. You are uninvolved in providing any type of care.
____	**3. Supportive:** You are concerned about the physical well-being of your loved one. You provide appropriate personal care freely and respectfully, but you maintain an emotional distance, as a professional would.
____	**4. Warmly supportive:** You are concerned about the physical as well as the emotional well-being of your loved one. You provide appropriate personal care freely and respectfully, with compassion and love, even though it is sometimes difficult.
____	**5. Occasionally over-involved:** You are warmly supportive of your loved one. Occasionally you sacrifice important parts of your own life, or take over certain aspects of your loved one's life that they, or others, could manage. At times, caregiving leaves you feeling very tired.

_____	**6. Often over-involved:** You are warmly supportive of your loved one, but view caregiving as a constant responsibility and set of tasks that you must perform at the expense of your own needs. You often feel exhausted because of providing care in isolation, with little or no support.
_____	**7. Usually/always over-involved:** You are supportive of your loved one, but you anxiously attend to your loved one's every need. As a result, you are devoting all your personal time to providing care. You are taking over certain aspects of your loved one's life that they, or others, should manage. You are chronically exhausted because of caregiving

©Partners on the Path 2022 www.PartnersonthePath.com

Replenish Your Energy Activity #1: Interpreting My Score

The choice of *#4 is considered a good balance point.* This item represents the center, a place at which you find the capacity to handle your caregiving responsibilities as a manageable part of the rest of your life.

If you chose *#1, #2, or #3, you are more detached from the situation* than other caregivers. You may have some personal issues that prevent you from connecting with your loved one, performing caregiving duties or helping your caregiving partners. You and other caregivers may disagree on what kind of care, or how much care your loved one needs.

If you chose *#5, #6, or #7, you are intensely involved in the caregiving role.* You may now or in the future experience depression, anxiety, or caregiver burnout. The higher your number, the greater your risk. You need to set aside more time for yourself. Find opportunities to step away from your caregiving role so you can regain a healthy balance in your life.

Achieving Better Balance

If your approach is causing problems for you or your caregiving partners, try some of these ideas:

- Ask others involved in caregiving to complete the self-assessment.

- Discuss the difficulties you are having with balancing caregiving with other aspects of your life.

- Describe how imbalance impacts you and ask how it impacts others.

- With others involved with you in family caregiving, identify new, more balanced ways to provide care.

- Try one or two ways to bring better balance into your caregiving and look to see how helpful the change is.

Replenish Your Energy Activity #2: Which resilience behaviors do I usually use?

Resilience Self-Reflection Resilience is the ability to navigate and recover from adversity with awareness, intention, and skill. Resilience develops naturally through healthy and meaningful connections, balanced self-care, and an open, engaged mind. Building resilience promotes positive energy.				
In the past 3 months, how often has this statement been true for you? 1 = Never or rarely 2 = Sometimes 3 = Often 4 = Always or almost always For each item, choose the number that best describes you.				
1. **Close, Supportive Relationships:** I have three or more close, supportive people in my life (i.e., we trust and know each other well AND we are there for each other in difficult times).	1	2	3	4
2. **Benefiting More than Just Oneself:** I strive to benefit more than just myself without depleting myself or imposing unwelcome efforts.	1	2	3	4
3. **Meaningful Connection:** I have a sense of connection to something vast or greater than myself, and it brings meaning to my life and I bring meaning to it (Examples: nature, art, community, a calling or discipline, spirituality, religion, creativity, a cause.)	1	2	3	4
4. **Physical Self-Care:** I am physically active for 30-60 minutes daily, sleep consistently and adequately, spend at least an hour in outdoor daylight, and eat a balanced and moderate diet mostly of wholesome, minimally processed foods.	1	2	3	4
5. **Stress Reduction Practice:** I participate in at least one practice to quiet my mind and body. *(Examples: deep breathing, time in nature, prayer, journaling, sensory grounding, meditation, yoga, tai chi, qigong, progressive muscle relaxation, autogenic training, biofeedback, imagery work.)*	1	2	3	4
6. **Flexible Thinking:** When I am going through a difficult time, I consider multiple perspectives on it as well as multiple options for responding to it.	1	2	3	4
7. **Self-confidence:** I trust myself, my intuition, and my abilities.	1	2	3	4
8. **Openness to Experience:** I welcome, seek, and enjoy experiences new to me.	1	2	3	4
9. **Workability:** I approach challenges as though I can work through them somehow.	1	2	3	4
10. **Awareness:** I notice the world around me, and I anticipate opportunities and challenges because of what I notice.	1	2	3	4
11. **History of Adaptive Coping with Adversity:** When I have faced adversities, I have found healthy and adaptive ways to work through them.	1	2	3	4
12. **Willingness:** When challenges arise, I face them and I do not deny them, ignore them, or use alcohol, other drugs, or self-harming behaviors to avoid or cope with them.	1	2	3	4
13. **Engagement:** I engage earnestly in one or more activities that offer a positive challenge, focus my attention, and deeply reward me. *(Examples: meaningful work, playing a musical instrument, dance, artistic expression, volunteering, sports, deep learning.)* Other activity/s:	1	2	3	4

14. Big Picture: I keep perspective on my challenges by considering the bigger picture. *(Examples: Looking beyond my challenges to consider the effects of strengths, supports, resources, opportunities, and privilege. Considering my challenges in the context of the adversity that others face. Considering the humor in life's challenges and absurdities. Looking for what I can learn from current and past challenges. Focusing on my character/principles/values.)*	1	2	3	4
Scoring: Add-up the numbers you chose for each item. **To interpret your score, see the following Scoring Guide.**	My score is: _____			
Source: *Adapted from Resilience Self-Reflection by Drew Weis, PhD, LP.* Used with permission.				

Scoring Guide: Reviewing My Overall Resilience	
<u>Score</u>	<u>Assessment</u>
38 or higher	You are *likely to view yourself as resilient.* Assuming your view is accurate, you are likely to thrive in the face of challenges and could serve as a strong support and role model for others.
22 – 37	You are *likely to view yourself as having adequate resilience, and you will likely do fine with most challenges.* Unless you are selling yourself short on your assessment, you have some room for enhancing your resilience. Read below to learn more.
21 or lower	You are *likely to view yourself as struggling or having limited options in the face of difficult challenges.* Lower scores sometimes reflect having some strengths but limited options. Low scores across items are common among people who have had few challenges early in life or have been overwhelmed by challenges early in life. History is not destiny! Read below for ways to enhance your resilience.

References

Handbook of Adult Resilience (2010) by John Reich, Alex Zautra, & John Stuart Hall

The Resiliency Advantage: Master Change, Thrive Under Pressure, and Bounce Back from Setbacks (2005) by Al Siebert

Replenish Your Energy Activity #3: What behaviors will I use to build my resilience?

My Action Plan for Building Resilience **Directions:** Read through items on the chart. Check those that you want to *keep doing* and those you'd like to *start to do or do more often*. If other resilience-building behaviors come to mind, write them in on the blank lines provided in each section.	Keep Doing	Start Doing Do More
Physical		
1. Exercise.		
2. Get adequate sleep and rest.		
3. Practice good hygiene and grooming; dress well.		
4. Use medicine as prescribed; limit alcohol.		
5. Avoid using drugs or tobacco.		
Nutritional		
1. Eat a balanced, healthy diet.		
2. Get and adequate intake of fluid.		
3. Avoid eating empty calories.		
4. Limit salt, saturated fat and trans fats.		
5. Snack on healthy foods.		
Medical		
1. Access quality health care.		
2. Get preventive screenings: E.g. Blood pressure, diabetes, eyes.		
3. Prevent injuries.		
4. Manage and rehab injuries that have occurred.		
5. Manage chronic health conditions.		

Replenish Your Energy Activity #3: What behaviors will I use to build my resilience?

My Action Plan for Building Resilience *Continued*	Keep Doing	Start Doing Do More
Psychological		
1. Think and do things to boost my confidence and self-belief.		
2. Think in optimistic ways and change pessimistic thoughts.		
3. Practice mindfulness.		
4. Use active problem-solving behavior.		
5. Identify my feelings and share my feelings with others.		
6. Persist in my efforts, even when encountering difficulty.		
7. Accept uncertainty and ambiguity.		
8. Use re-labeling to help mentally cope with difficulties.		
9. Use physical activity to work-off intense emotions.		
Social		
1. Reach out to people and groups who provide positive support: Emotional, informational and/or hands-on-help.		
2. Participate in groups that offer support: In-person groups, online or telephone support groups.		
3. Try to imitate the lives and actions of inspiring individuals.		
4. Enjoy fun activities, hobbies, and socializing with others.		
5. Take time-off from doing work of any kind, and time to be alone.		
6. If employed outside the home, mentally separate work and home.		

Environmental		
1. Recognize and address environmental stressors: • Temperature		
• Noise and interruptions		
• Air quality.		
2. Take measures to assure safety in my home or workplace.		
3. Take measures to prevent injuries in my home or workplace.		
4. Avoid taking unnecessary risks.		
5. Do things to organize or beautify my home or workplace.		
Spiritual		
1. Identify the values, beliefs and purpose that give my life meaning.		
2. Regularly connect with God or what gives my life meaning.		
3. Regularly pray, worship or meditate.		
4. Enjoy experiences of nature or the arts.		
5. Read texts, watch shows, and listen to music that is inspiring.		

© Partners on the Path 2022. www.PartnersonthePath.com

Helpful Resources

American Psychological Association: Building Your Resilience https://www.apa.org/topics/resilience provides trustworthy guidance on why and how to become more resilient.

Caring for the Caregiver: Center yourself https://youtu.be/tblc5QoOLsQ YouTube video from the author on how to conserve and replenish your energy.

Caregiver Concerns: Overwhelmed
https://www.youtube.com/watch?v=nCxJRvomrbc

Gawain, Shakti. *The Four Levels of Healing: A Guide to Balancing the Spiritual, Mental, Emotional and Physical Aspects of Life.* New World Library. 1997

Gawain, Shakti. *Creative Visualization*. New World Library. 2016.

McCleod, Beth Witrogen. *Caregiving: The Spiritual Journey of Love, Loss and Renewal.* John Wiley & Sons. 2000.

One Moment Meditation: Martin Boroson https://www.youtube.com/watch?v=F6eFFCi12v8 this animated video introduces a technique that allows you to meditate whenever you want to…One-Moment Meditation.

Remen, Rachel Naomi. *Kitchen Table Wisdom: Stories that Heal. Tenth Anniversary Edition.* Riverhead Books. 2006.

Schaef, Anne Wilson. *Meditations for Women Who Do Too Much. Revised Edition.* Harper Collins. 2004.

"The real man smiles in trouble, gathers strength from distress, and grows brave by reflection."
Thomas Paine
American revolutionary leader; author of *Common Sense*

"The highest levels of performance come to people who are centered, intuitive, creative, and reflective - people who know to see a problem as an opportunity."
Deepak Chopra
Indian-American author and alternative-medicine advocate

"Serenity is not freedom from the storm, but peace amid the storm."
Debenport
Unknown

CHAPTER 8

Self-Care: Think Optimistically

Jane's Story: Pennies on My Path

I am drowning! My husband is in constant pain. Dad is going blind and can hardly breathe. Mother is losing her mind. My mother-in-law had a stroke and can't care for herself anymore. I have a four-year-old son who never stops moving, and I just moved into a house that polite people would call a fixer-upper. The stress is getting to be so much that I wonder if I will lose my mind, too. My life feels like such a wreck; I'm even dreaming about debris.

Last week I dreamed I was walking on a rainy, windy night. My coat collar pulled up and my head down, I was leaning into the blustery, bitter wind. Looking down at the sodden leaves and dirt in the gutter, something caught my eye. I bent to see more clearly what it was. There in the puddle atop some muddy decaying leaves, I found a shiny penny. Into my mind popped the old saying, "Find a penny pick it up and all day long you'll have good luck." Then I noticed more coins among the rubbish in the gutter: nickels, dimes, and quarters! I felt ecstatic, and then abruptly woke. Lying in bed, for some reason I smiled and felt happy. Trash and cash in the gutter, what could this mean?

The following evening a remarkable thing happened. While walking after dinner to clear my mind, I was deep in thought, head down, when something caught my eye. I leaned over to see what it was. There among the leaves and dirt in the road near my house was a penny! Returning home from my walk that night I smiled and felt happy like after my dream. Amazingly, in the past five days I have found four more coins in the road, and they each filled me with some inexplicable delight.

Being happy about pennies makes no logical sense, yet every time I find one I am reassured. There are many ways of interpreting my dream, but I feel as if God is talking to me through these coins, encouraging me during these tough times. He seems to be saying, "You can see me amidst the rubble in your life; just look closely and keep walking. Your life may seem to be in the gutter, but some shining moments are mixed in. I will help in ways you might overlook, because they may seem as small and insignificant as a penny. But I will provide just what you need no matter what the circumstances of your life."

Are you finding pennies on your path?

Are you walking through a difficult or dark part of life? Are you finding pennies or some other talisman as you journey on? When my life was turned upside down, I struggled to remain optimistic and find something positive among so many painful circumstances. The pennies on my path raised my spirits and helped me to see the mixture of good and bad in my life. How are you viewing your life right now? One powerful way to remain optimistic in the face of caregiving challenges is to think in positive ways…and look for some "pennies" of you own!

Self-Care Recommendations

What are optimism and pessimism?

Optimism and pessimism are the lenses through which you look at the world. They color the stories you create to explain events. Whether you realize it or not, these stories are active thought patterns that you control. They become habits that determine how you respond to life events, who you become and how others respond to you.

How do pessimists think?

Pessimists think *positive events are unlikely to happen again, and that negative ones are likely to continue* or be repeated in the future. They believe that *good situations are isolated events or flukes* that have nothing to do with other aspects of their lives. In contrast, they think negative circumstances are experienced in many aspects of their lives and *expect that more of the same negative experiences are inevitable.* Finally, pessimists believe that *good outcomes are <u>brought about by others</u> or other factors beyond their control,* and the bad outcomes are usually their own fault. Pessimists *emphasize the negative no matter what the facts of the situation.*

How do optimists think?

Optimists think in the opposite way. They *view positive events as likely to continue or be repeated in the future and negative ones as unlikely to happen again.* They believe that *good situations are experienced in many aspects of their lives;* more of the same are inevitable. On the other hand, *negative events are isolated or are flukes* that have nothing to do with other aspects of their lives. Finally, optimists *believe <u>they</u> bring about good outcomes and think the bad ones are caused by others,* or by other factors beyond their control. Optimists *emphasize the positive no matter what the facts of the situation.*

What are the benefits of being an optimist?

If you adopt an optimistic outlook, you are likely to experience:

1. *Strength to handle adversity*: to persevere and adapt in times of trouble.

2. *Decreased stress*: a positive frame of mind, more success, and less mental strain.

3. *Good physical and emotional health*: positive mood and morale; aging well & experiencing fewer physical ills.

4. *Successful relationships*: others react well to a contagious, positive outlook.

How can I become more optimistic?

1. *Choose to change*: Pessimistic patterns remain in place until *you choose* to replace these negative practices with positive ones.

2. *Stop and listen to your thoughts*: Pay attention. As soon as a negative thought comes to you, replace it with a positive one. The more you *challenge negative thinking and reinforce your positive thoughts*, the more automatic optimism will become.

   Don't be a Pollyanna: Being *unrealistic optimists*, Pollyanna's unwisely plunge ahead, ignoring real needs or threats that can increase their stress and risk of health problems. *Choose realistic optimism*, a lens that promotes clear thinking. *Realistic or cautious optimists*:

   • Have a positive outlook *without denying reality*.

   • Appreciate positive elements in a situation, *while also acknowledging the negative*.

- Hope for positive outcomes *without assuming good results will automatically occur.*

- Accomplish positive outcomes *with hard work, planning and effective problem solving.*

3. *Affirm yourself*: Affirmations are *words, brief phrases or sentences that reprogram your mind to more optimistically see, explain and respond to situations in your life.* Affirming yourself is really quite simple.

Choose an event or behavior: a *positive one to encourage, or negative one to eliminate.* Choose words carefully. For a *positive*: Describe it as caused by you, likely to continue and affecting your entire life. For a *negative*: Describe it as an isolated incident, not your fault and unlikely to occur again.

Affirm this as the reality in your life, right now. Use *first-person and present tense to imagine this as a reality you are experiencing now.* For example, "I am capable, confident and compassionate. I find meaning and joy in being a caregiver." Select *words that are vivid, and that stir up positive feeli*ngs within. *Write affirmations and post them* where you will see them throughout the day.

Regularly repeat positive affirmations *silently or aloud, until you know them by heart.* Savor the positive image and feelings the affirmation creates. Frequent repetition reprograms your mind.

4. **Visualize**: Visualization is *daydreaming with the positive purpose of relieving stress, overcoming obstacles, or becoming more optimistic.* Follow these three guidelines.

Vividly picture a positive scene in your mind's eye like vacationing on a tropical island, completing a marathon, or experiencing a joyous birthday or holiday celebration. *Use all your senses*: sight, hearing, taste, touch and smell. Detail is most important. *The more vivid the image, the more helpful it will be.*

Envision this as the reality in your life, right now. Create images in the *first-person and present tense* to picture this as a reality you are experiencing now.

Savor that scene for several moments, several times each day. You can visualize virtually *anywhere,* but in bed each morning and just before sleep at night are relaxed, easy times to practice visualization. Choose a time that works best for you. *Regular visualization actually creates your new reality.*

5. ***Avoid pessimism in the world around you***: *Emotions are contagious.* Take a break from violent images, depressing stories, and people who are downbeat. Seek out people and situations that create positive energy and reinforce positive messages for you.

6. ***Contain the damages***: *When negative events do occur, create an optimistic explanation in your mind.* Think of all the extenuating circumstances that might have created the negative events. Name what outside circumstances contributed to this situation. Remember that problems in a given instance neither suggest nor confirm your personal weakness. Remind yourself that there will be many opportunities to do better in the future.

Activities for Caregivers

Think Optimistically Activity #1: How optimistic am I?

> **Revised Life Orientation Test (LOT-R)**
> Directions: Read through the ten descriptions below. Use the following scale to identify your response for each item.
>   0 = Strongly Disagree
>   1 = Disagree
>   2 = Neutral
>   3 = Agree
>   4 = Strongly Disagree
> Please be as honest and accurate as possible. Try not to let your response to one statement influence your responses to other statements. There are no "correct" or "incorrect" answers. Answer according to your own feelings, rather than how you think "most people" would answer.

1. In uncertain times, I usually expect the best.	
2. It's easy for me to relax.	
3. If something can go wrong for me it will.	
4. I'm always optimistic about my future.	
5. I enjoy my friends a lot.	
6. It's important for me to keep busy.	
7. I hardly ever expect things to go my way.	
8. I don't get upset too easily.	
9. I rarely count on good things happening to me.	
10. Overall, I expect more good things to happen to me than bad.	

Calculating Your Score

1. **Reverse code items 3, 7 and 9. Change your answers for these items:**

   Score of 0; change it to 4
   Score of 1; change it to 3
   Score of 2 remains a 2
   Score of 3; change it to 1
   Score of 4; change it to 0

2. **Total up items 1, 3, 4, 9, and 10 to obtain your overall score: _____**

3. **Items 2, 5, 6, and 8 are filler items only. They do not contribute to your LOT-R score.**

Interpreting Your Score

Your score could range from 0-24. The higher your score and the closer it is to 24, the more optimistic in outlook you are.

- **A total score of 0-5** indicates that you are highly pessimistic and low on optimism.

- **A total score of 14-18** indicates that you are moderately optimistic.

- **A total score of 19-24** indicates that you are highly optimistic and low on pessimism.

Source: Carver, C. S. (2013) Life Orientation Test-Revised (LOT-R). Measurement Instrument Database for the Social Science.

Think Optimistically Activity #2: What affirmation could help me?

Affirmation Action Plan
Follow the three steps below to create and use a helpful affirmation in your life.
Step 1: Choose either 1 or 2 listed below and **describe what you are trying to create** in your life. Write your response in the space below or on a separate piece of paper. 1. The **positive** event, behavior, attitude or trait I want to **encourage** is… 　*E.g. I want to be patient and calm when my Mother repeatedly asks the same question.* 2. The **negative** event, behavior, attitude or trait I want to **eliminate** is… 　*E.g. I don't want to blow up and argue when talking with my siblings about Mom's needs.*

Step 2: Using the five guidelines listed below, **create the affirmation** as if it already part of your life. Record your affirmation by completing this sentence: "My affirmation is…"
1. Use **first-person**: Start the affirmation with "I".
2. Use **present-tense**: Select words that say it is already true, a reality you are experiencing now, not something you wish to have or hope for in the future.
3. Use **positive** words: Generate upbeat feelings within yourself.
4. Use **vivid** words: Paint a clear picture that you can see, feel, and hear.
5. Use **realistic** images: Choose hopeful, positive pictures that seem right for you.

E.g. I am patient when Mom asks the same questions over and over. Because I love her, I answer calmly and accept that she is doing the best she can.
E.g. I discuss Mom's needs calmly, respectfully and assertively. I am comfortable with the outcome of our discussion.

Step 3: Select **ways to remind you** of your affirmation.
- Regularly repeat the affirmation aloud or silently each morning when you rise, or each evening when you go to bed.
- Write your affirmation on top of your to-do list, on post-it notes or 3x5 cards that you place in prominent places.

Think Optimistically Activity #3: What visualization could help me?

Visualization Action Plan
Follow the three steps below to create your own visual image and use it to care for yourself.

Step 1: Choose either 1 or 2 listed below and **describe what you are trying to create** in your life. Write your response in the space below or on a separate piece of paper.
    1.   Do I seek some **relief from the stress** in my life? E.g. I feel overwhelmed by stress and just want to relax.
    2.   Do I want to overcome **a specific obstacle**? E.g. I don't want to blow up at my siblings about Mom's needs.

Step 2: Use these four guidelines & envision the scene as if it's already part of your life. Record your visualization below.

1. Use **first-person**: Picture yourself in the image.
2. Use **present-tense**: Imagine that this picture is a reality you are experiencing right now.
3. Use **positive images**: Generate upbeat feelings within yourself by seeing things you like and that feel good to you.
   The more positive, the more helpful it will be.
4. Use **vivid images**: Paint a detailed picture using all five senses, including elements that you clearly can see, feel, taste, smell and hear. The more vivid, the more helpful it will be.

E.g. **To relieve stress:** *I am lying on the beach on a tropical island. The air temperature is a warm 80 degrees; a gentle breeze is blowing in from the ocean. The warm, bright sun is sparkling off the turquoise water. I hear the waves rolling in and the sea gulls calling as they dive down and catch fish just off shore. Little shore birds are skittering up the beach just ahead of the incoming wave. Calypso music is being played on a metal drum and a trio of men is melodiously singing island songs. I am sipping a cool, refreshing pina colada, leaning back on my beach chair and wiggling my toes in the warm sand. My muscles are relaxed and I am holding my beloved's hand as we gaze on the children frolicking in the waves, squealing with delight. As I breathe in, I feel calm and at peace.*

E.g. **To overcome my negative feelings and handle a difficult situation:** *I am sitting with my brother and sister at my kitchen table. In a calm, respectful tone I ask John and Emily to visit Mom more frequently. When they begin to offer excuses why they cannot do this, I inhale slowly and deeply. I feel relaxation in my chest and shoulders. I hear them accuse me of not understanding and feel a warm protective shield form around me. Their criticisms are deflected and bounce off like little rubber balls that fly off into space. They look funny and make me smile. I see myself drinking warm, sweet nectar that fills me with a sense of strength from within. I have the right response to whatever John or Emily say. My words are assertive, respectful and calm. They listen and hear my perspective. Our discussion resolves the disagreement. Mom is well cared for.*

Step 3: Savor that scene for several moments, several times each day. You can visualize virtually anywhere, but in bed each morning or before sleep at night are relaxed times to practice visualization. Choose a time that works best for you.

Think Optimistically Activity #4: Guided Self-Reflection

My Thoughts: Guided Self-Reflection
Directions: Use the following questions to help you explore your optimism and consider ways that you could expand it.
1. Small Signs of Encouragement
Name It • In Jane's Story, pennies are the talisman that spoke to her of hope in times of trouble. What sign or symbol of encouragement and support am I noticing? What affect does it have on me?
2. My Thoughts
Name It • In what one caregiving situation could I practice being more optimistic? • At present, what are my thoughts that are pessimistic or negative? • What positive thoughts could I use to replace these?

3. Pollyanna's

<u>Name It</u>
- What fictional character or real person do I know that is a Pollyanna?
- Am I a Pollyanna? If so, what are some of the consequences I have suffered as a result of unrealistic optimism?
- How can I be more realistic about my expectations?

4. Avoiding Toxicity

<u>Name It</u>
- Where or when do I experience violent images, toxic behaviors, or downbeat situations?
- How do these impact me and how can I protect myself from these?

Helpful Resources

Authentic Happiness: https://www.authentichappiness.sas.upenn.edu/testcenter offers positive psychology questionnaires and resources from The Positive Psychology Center at the University of Pennsylvania. On-line questionnaires provide feedback on character strengths and virtues, happiness, optimism, satisfaction with life, and related positive psychology topics while providing the university with confidential responses for online research studies.

Ban Breathnach, Sarah. *Simple Abundance: A Daybook of Comfort and Joy*. Hachette Book Group. 2019.

Gratefulness: https://gratefulness.org/ is an international nonprofit organization that provides resources for living courageously and gratefully, despite life circumstances. Their broad mission and array of resources promote reconciliation and healing for individuals, relationships and the world.

Lyubomirsky, Sonja. *The How of Happiness: A New Approach to Getting the Life You Want*. Penguin Books. 2008.

Seligman, Martin. *Learned Optimism: How to Change Your Mind and Your Life*. Vintage. 2011.

You'll be Okay https://vimeo.com/18023045 video of the author telling the story that opens this chapter.

"Gratitude unlocks the fullness of life. It turns what we have into enough, and more. It turns denial into acceptance, chaos to order, confusion to clarity. It can turn a meal into a feast, a house into a home, a stranger into a friend."
Melody Beattie
Self-help author who popularized the concept of co-dependence

"Optimism is the madness of insisting that all is well when we are miserable."
Voltaire
French philosopher

"The essence of optimism is that it takes no account of the present, but it is a source of inspiration, of vitality and hope where others have resigned. It enables a man to hold his head high, to claim the future for himself and not to abandon it to his enemy."
Dietrich Bonhoeffer
Theologian hanged for plot against Hitler

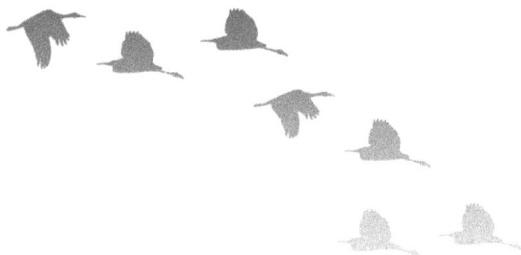

CHAPTER 9

Self-Care: Choose Wisely

Jane's Story: Think about your choices!

One day when my son Rob was a third grader, I went to his school for a visit. His classmates were returning from after-lunch recess, still exploding with wild energy and earsplitting "playground" voices. The din reverberated through the school hallway as Rob's teacher, Mrs. Wilson, and I came around the corner. The children didn't see either of us, but they snapped to attention when they heard Mrs. Wilson loudly clap her hands three times. Then, in a commanding, yet calm and caring tone, she called out, "Students, think about your choices and make sure they are good ones!" What a teacher!

With those few words, she transformed a pack of young ruffians into angels! The third graders quieted, formed two lines, and walked silently into their classroom. They settled into their desks and began to focus on the work at hand. If I had not seen it, I would not have believed that Mrs. Wilson's instructions could make such a difference. It was amazing!

Now, eight years later I am thinking of Mrs. Wilson's words: *"Think about your choices and make sure they're good ones!"* I wish those words could so easily transform my life, but I am not in the third grade. Instead of energetic playmates pushing me, it is an overwhelming list of parent-spouse-worker-caregiver responsibilities that feel like a stick poking me in the back, relentlessly driving me on. Worries about how to help both Mom and Dad from so many miles away scream out and wake me in the night. Imaginary scenarios of telling off people who bungle my parents' care are proxies for my yelling at God. How *could* He let Mother lose her mind and Dad lose his sight?!! The third graders were out of hand in a sweet, youthful way; I am out of control in a tormented way.

The kids knew what to choose to get back on track; the tone of Mrs. Wilson's voice made it completely clear. Sometimes I don't know what to choose. Move Mom to the dementia unit or keep her at home? Confront a problem or let it go? Tough it out or take the antidepressant? So much of what is happening is beyond my control: my parents' health and decline; my feelings of sadness and loss; how far away I live from my folks; how much I need to be home with my husband and yet long to be with Mom and Dad. I need to think about my choices and make sure they are healthy ones.

What kind of choices are you making?

As a caregiver you are confronted with many difficult and often painful choices. When making these caregiving choices, ask yourself the following questions about *what you are choosing* and *how you are making your choice.*

Self-Care Recommendations

Is this a healthy choice?

A wise choice is *never one that undermines your health or the health of others*. Health is being sound or whole, free from disease or pain in body, mind, or soul. If your choice *fosters well-being* in any of these areas, it likely is a very good choice.

Healthy choices also *promote balance in your life*. Each of us has a limited supply of resources: energy, time, patience, knowledge, money. Like an overdrawn bank account, living beyond the limits of your resources is unhealthy. So recognize your limits and make sure your choices are made with them in mind. Wise choices *simplify rather than complicate your life*.

Is this a loving choice?

A wise choice is *never one that undermines human dignity and worth*. Loving choices are made with an *attitude of appreciation*. They lead to caring acts that acknowledge worth, address needs, or nurture growth in you or in others. Wise caregiving choices *acknowledge and respect the needs of both the caregiver and the care receiver*. By caring for yourself as you care for others, you model balance and show that helping others can be a meaningful and loving choice. Wise caregiving choices send this encouraging message to all those who work with you, who witness and learn from your caregiving efforts.

Is this a "big rock"?

A wise choice is *never one that loses sight of what is most vital*. In Stephen Covey's work and many website postings, there is the story of a teacher standing before a group of students. Into a large clear jar are poured big rocks, then smaller pebbles to fill in the spaces. Asked if the jar is full, the class answers, "Yes." The students see they are wrong when the teacher adds sand and finally water. The restricted capacity of the jar limits how much it can hold. By starting with the big rocks the teacher fits more in than anyone could have imagined. The moral of the story: "Put the big rocks in first!"

Like the jar, *you have restricted capacity; there is just so much you can take.* Big rocks are the most significant things in life; things that are good for the health of your body, heart, mind and soul. Pebbles are valuable but less critical. The sand and water are fun, trivial or unnecessary aspects that may be nice but are not essential. In your life, you define what are big rocks and sand. You *need self-awareness to discover the limits of your capacity, and your important values and priorities.* Spending time on what is unimportant is like filling the jar with sand and water first, a poor choice because it may leave no time for what is truly vital. A wise choice is one that *recognizes your limits and helps you spend time on what is most important.*

Would this choice pass the "death-bed" test?

Wise choices *yield outcomes that stand the test of time.* When trying to make difficult choices, it is tough to maintain a clear perspective and be sure of the best choice. By *focusing on a long-term perspective and on your priorities*, the "death-bed" question helps you sort things out. Picture yourself lying on your death-bed, preparing to breathe your last. What would you think of your choice in that situation? Rooted in the values that are truly important to you, the "death-bed" question will help you choose wisely.

Am I letting others choose for me?

Faced with a dilemma or decision, you have no choice but to choose. You may make a decision on your own or in consultation with others. You may decide now, later, or not decide at all. Even if you opt not to make a choice, the situation unfolds. Inaction allows outside forces to select for you and create outcomes that may or may not work in your favor. When you let others choose, you run the risk of their making selections that don't fit with your values, satisfy your needs or promote your well-being.

Exercising choice is a powerful way to create the life you want to live. Don't give this power away to others. If you are fearful, do something to bolster your courage. Take as much time as you have; don't rush. Use both the intelligence of your mind and the understanding of your heart to help you choose wisely.

Am I being honest?

About the facts: Facing the facts is a key component of choosing wisely, even if you don't like the facts. *Avoidance, distortion, denial and entitlement are mental tricks that deflect attention from painful realities.* Face the facts.

About my responsibilities: The behavior you choose and decisions you make have consequences that shape your life and create your reality. *Don't blame other people for difficulties in your life.* Acknowledging your responsibilities and choosing wisely can sometimes demand great courage and personal strength. When you take responsibility for your life, your choices will serve you well. Take responsibility for yourself.

About my viewpoint: Finally, it is wise to be honest about your perspective on people and situations. *Don't mistake your views for objective truth. They are not. Your perspective is just one way of interpreting reality.* Others have different perspectives and they are just as valid as yours. Always *check your viewpoint against real data* to find the truth in a situation. Wise choices flow from an accurate grasp of reality. Acknowledge that your point of view is subjective.

Can I let go?

All of life cycles through seasons; nothing stays the same forever. When people or practices, habits or attitudes that once were life giving cease to serve your needs, holding on generates distress. Look closely to identify old patterns or relationships that undermine your well-being. It is wise to *hold onto what gives meaning to your life, and to let go of relationships or routines that no longer sustain you.*

Letting go can also be a choice to forgive. Forgiveness *is not* condoning, absolving, forgetting or self-sacrifice. It is not a clear-cut, one-time decision. Forgiveness *is* a process of moving beyond feelings about people or past incidents and releasing grudges, resentment or self-pity. It involves putting the past in proper perspective, and giving up the desire to punish others or yourself for past actions. Choosing to let go allows you to reclaim energy for healing and moving on to more positive life experiences.

Activities for Caregivers

Choose Wisely Activity #1: What healthy self-care practices do I usually use?

Self-Care Checklist: Self-care is a healthy choice. Check your current practices and some you'll begin using. Aim for diversity and frequency in self-care; it's best for your health!		
Physical		
-- Exercise regularly -- Rest during the day -- Sleep 7-8 hours at night -- Eat a balanced diet -- Limit "junk food" -- Drink eight glasses of water daily	-- Maintain weight in desired range -- Limit alcohol consumption -- Do not smoke -- Use medications as prescribed __ Visit physician for check-ups __ Practice yoga	-- Practice the relaxation response -- Groom yourself – manicure, facial, haircut, shave, etc. -- Get a massage __ Receive chiropractic care __ Practice Reiki __ Engage in outdoor activities
Emotional		
-- Allow yourself to feel emotions -- Appropriately & respectfully express emotions -- Work off anger with physical exercise -- Say "no" when you want or need to -- Ask directly for what you want	-- Cry -- Laugh -- Resolve conflicts -- Nurture yourself -- Don't take things too seriously	
Mental		
-- Ask questions -- Accept ambiguity -- Read -- Take risks __ Practice guided imagery	-- Daydream -- Learn something new -- Consider different viewpoints -- Read self-help books __ Use visualization or affirmation	-- Relabel unpleasant situations -- Develop plans -- Think optimistically -- Use helpful web-based resources __ Take responsibility for yourself/your life
Social		
-- Develop and use support systems -- Talk with friends and family -- Take time off -- Go on vacation -- Rehabilitate or end unsatisfactory relationships -- Limit TV viewing -- Engage in a creative pastime or hobby	-- Read humorous books/watch humorous shows -- Socialize with others -- Enjoy intimacy or sex -- Play -- Spend time alone -- Treat yourself to something enjoyable: new clothes, CD's, magazine, etc. -- Engage in volunteer activities	

Spiritual		
–– Pray or meditate –– Commune with nature –– "Let go" of unsolvable problems	–– Attend worship services –– Read inspirational prose or poetry –– Appreciate the beauty of art or music	–– Take one day at a time –– Clarify your values and beliefs –– Acknowledge your self-worth

Occupational: Employment and/or Caregiving Work	
–– Learn new skills –– Pace yourself –– Balance involvement and detachment –– Seek respite-daily, periodic, short term, or vacations –– Get organized –– Take breaks –– Do your best and let go of the rest	–– Share responsibilities with others –– Let others sometimes do a stressful/difficult task –– Beautify your environment –– Acknowledge the good you do –– Leave work at work –– Develop good relationships with co-workers –– Open yourself to change __ Use Employee Assistance Program/your employer's helpful resources

Problem Solving Action	
__ Effectively manage time __ Assertively communicate with others __ Negotiate with others for desired outcomes __ Constructively resolve conflict __ Create a comfortable home	__ Learn new information or life skills __ Change dysfunctional/self-defeating behaviors __ Clarify or resolve misunderstandings __ Budget and wisely manage finances __ Keep possessions in good working order

©Partners on the Path. 2022. www.PartnersonthePath.com

Choose Wisely Activity #2: Guided Self-Reflection

Letting Go: Guided Self-Reflection

Directions: Read the following poem to help you reflect on your feelings about letting go of situations that no longer give energy, joy, purpose or meaning to your life. Then answer the following questions.

To "Let Go" Takes Love (Author Unknown)

To "Let Go" does not mean to stop caring.
It means I can't do it for someone else.
To "Let Go" is not to enable,
but to allow learning from natural consequences.
To "Let Go" is to admit powerlessness,
which means the outcome is not in my hands.
To "Let Go" is not to care for, but to care about.
To "Let Go" is not to fix, but to be supportive.
To "Let Go" is not to judge,
but to allow another to be himself or herself.
To "Let Go" is not to be in the middle arranging all the outcomes,
but to allow others to determine their own destinies.
To "Let Go" is not to be less protective,
it is to permit another to face reality.
To "Let Go" is not to dominate,
but to be willing to let things happen.
To "Let Go" is to not to betray the past,
but to have faith in the future.
To "Let Go" means to fear less and to love more.

- What responsibilities, people, thought patterns, behaviors, habits, or living arrangements do you need to *let go*? How are you currently *holding on* to these situations?

- How do you feel about *letting go*?

- Do you need some help letting go? Who could help you?

- What action on your part would help you to *let go*?

- What benefits might you receive if you *let go*?

Choose Wisely Activity #3: Guided Self-Reflection

My Caregiving Decisions: Guided Self-Reflection
Directions: Use the following questions to help you explore how you make caregiving decisions and how you could improve.
1. As a caregiver, what are my biggest decisions or most difficult choices? What makes them so big or difficult?
2. What are the best and the worst caregiving decisions I ever made? What made them so? Are there lessons I learned that could be applied to future choices?
3. Who are people on whom I can rely when faced with difficult choices in these areas: • Health care: • Insurance: • Finances: • Legal matters: • Household management: • Handling emotions:

4. What are some healthy and some unhealthy choices I have made for myself? How did these affect my family or friends? Would I make the same choices in the future? If so, why? If not, why not?

5. Are there times when I avoid choosing or let others choose for me? What are the results, either positive or negative, that are associated with "choosing not to choose?"

6. What are the "big rocks" in my life, the values and priorities I need to honor when I make choices?

7. What are difficult caregiving responsibilities I'd rather avoid, deny or change? Which of my personal perspectives do I treat as if they were objective fact? What are the consequences of being less than honest with myself?

Helpful Resources

Allen, James. *As You Think: A Reworking of As A Man Thinketh*. Inspiration Revisited. 2020.

Bridges, William and Susan. *Managing Transitions: Making the Most of Change. 25ᵗʰ anniversary edition*. DaCapo Lifelong Books. 2017.

Caring for the Caregiver: Choose Wisely https://www.youtube.com/watch?v=X6v4Q5KZO-E&t=6s a YouTube video from the author with ideas on how to make difficult choices.

Covey, Stephen. *The 7 Habits of Highly Effective People: 30ᵗʰ Anniversary Edition*. Simon & Schuster. 2020.

Douty, Linda. *How Can I Let Go if I Don't Know I'm Holding On?* Morehouse Publishing. 2005.

Fear of Transformation, written by Danaan Parry, is a brief, inspirational story about change and transition. It can be found on the web in print: http://www.earthstewards.org/ESN-Trapeze.asp and as a YouTube video: https://www.youtube.com/watch?v=HWvV5N4hOGc

Green, Eboni Ivory. *At the Heart of the Matter: A Self-Help Workbook for Caregivers.* Self-published. 2021.

"Forgiveness does not change the past but it does enlarge the future."
Paul Boese
Dutch botanist, known for famous quotes

"We can choose to wake up and grumble all day and be bitter and angry and judge others and find satisfaction in others doing bad instead of good. Or we can we wake up with optimism and love and say, 'Just what is this beautiful day going to bring me?'"
Margaret Trudeau
Canadian author and activist

"Realize deeply that the present moment is all you ever have. Make the Now the primary focus of your life."
Eckhart Tolle
Spiritual teacher and author of *The Power of Now*

CHAPTER 10

Self-Care: Connect With Care Partners

Jane's Story: Why won't you walk with me?

I don't understand why some of my closest friends and family seem to be AWOL: absent without leave during these desperate days. Maybe they don't recognize my desperation. Dad unexpectedly died within hours of having a stroke 10 months ago, on Mother's Day. Mom's dementia has gotten much worse since then. A small group of steadfast souls still see Mom since Dad's death, but most have stopped visiting. Few call to offer support, and some don't even ask how things are going. Maybe they don't want to know.

Why am I so angry? Everyone is busy. People may not know what to say. Some family members have been distant for years. I shouldn't expect anything different now, but I guess I do. I want family and friends I can depend on for support. I long for relationships that feel life giving like oxygen.

I am really hurt, as well as angry. I feel let down. I would like to be able to turn to others for help to get through these horrors called dementia and death. Sometimes, when there is no specific task that can be done, I simply could use a hug from a loving person. In times of crisis isn't it natural to turn to our family and friends for support? Don't I have a right to be disappointed and mad?

Do you ever feel disconnected from the support of family or friends?

Although I had a right to feel disappointed and mad, it was a huge waste of time and energy. It took buckets of tears and more than a year's time after my Mother's death to see that I was looking for help where it could not be found. For many reasons, some of my friends and family were not there for me when I really needed them.

How about you? Are you in dire need of support? Do you have a circle of family and friends who are there for you in times of need? The caregiving experience showed me the importance of cultivating a diverse community who would sustain me when life is difficult. It taught me that clinging to my wants and expectations, and asking "Why?" causes problems. I learned another lesson the hard way. Asking for help from someone who hasn't got it to give is as futile as trying to find milk in an egg carton.

Self-Care Recommendations

Why is connecting with others so important?

As a human being, you are a social animal, wired for relating to other people. You gain strength and energy from connecting with your spouse or other family members; with friends, neighbors or people in your faith community. The positive benefits that come from cultivating a supportive community include:

1. **Improved health**: reduced stress, more resilience and a stronger immune system.

2. **Richer resources**: access to helpful information, skills, talents assets or energy.

3. **Smarter choices**: consultation and reassurance when decisions are difficult.

4. **Better balance**: energy for "juggling" or help from others who will relieve you of demands.

5. **Deeper appreciation**: ability to face dilemmas and see both the good and the bad.

What can I do to connect with others?

Picture the community around you as a well-stocked refrigerator that is filled with food to sustain you. Healthy caregivers strike a balance between doing their work and preserving their capacity to care. Energy flows out when providing care; that energy needs to be replenished. Refuel your body and soul with help from those who surround you.

1. **Open the door**: Like a well-stocked refrigerator in the heart of your home, the refreshment you so need to continue caring is there for you, if you just open the door. *Go to your friends and family to be fed.*

2. **Feast on healthy food, as well as on a few treats**. Think about *your needs*, what would relieve your stress or solve some of your caregiving problems. Also think of *your wants*; what would simply be fun and pleasing to do with a friend or family member. In life as in caregiving, sometimes we need a full meal; sometimes we just want a cookie. *Look to your friends and family for both.*

3. **Feed yourself—ask for what you need.** When your body needs food you don't wait for others to guess if you are hungry. You don't criticize yourself for being hungry. You open the refrigerator door and get some food. So as a caregiver, *don't passively wait for others to guess your needs, or apologize for having needs.* Ask others to help with caregiving tasks or managing your own affairs that, because of caregiving responsibilities, have become too much to handle. *Be specific, direct and respectful when you ask for help.*

4. **Let others feed you**. *Don't always try to do things yourself.* Take in energy from the community of friends and family who support you. *If accepting help is difficult, remember how good it feels to give.* In receiving, you offer others an opportunity to affirm their generosity and express their love. *Graciously accept help that is offered, in whatever form it takes.*

5. **Choose dependable brands**. Your support system is like the contents of your refrigerator; some brands and some people deliver the goods better than others. *Go to those who will deliver real support*: those who are reliable and concerned about you; optimistic and hopeful, yet realistic; people who can listen and help you make good decisions. *Avoid negative or self-centered people who make you feel guilty or uncomfortable for needing help.*

6. **Look for milk in the milk carton, not in the egg carton.** You know it is absurd to look for milk among the eggs. *Don't waste your energy seeking help from people who are unable or unwilling*

to provide what you need. Seek support from those who want to support you. Also, *ask others to do things that they like, are good at, or feel comfortable doing.* This approach increases the likelihood of actually receiving the help you need, and allows those who give to feel good about doing something for you.

7. **Go to the pitcher that is full, not the one that's empty.** Seeking support from folks who are tapped out or over committed is as unsatisfying as trying to get a glass of juice from an empty pitcher. *Look for help from people who have a bit more time or balance in their lives.* Also, *don't be too quick to judge* those who are over extended. They have a right to choose how they spend their time; you do not own their lives…they do. Accept the reality of others' limitations. *Empty pitchers are empty. Being upset won't fill them up.*

8. **Restock the refrigerator.** Just as the refrigerator runs low on food without a replenishing trip to the market, *relationships with those in your support system get depleted without your giving something back.* Tending relationships refills the reservoir of good will that inspires your supporters to help during difficult times. How do you restock? Here are some ideas you might find helpful:

    - *Express gratitude.* Say "thank you" in person, by phone, email or writing a note of thanks.

    - *Demonstrate genuine interest.* Ask about what is happening in the other's life; listen to their response.

    - *Show kindness and respect.* Speak and act in ways that show you care. Treat others as you would like to be treated.

    - *Keep commitments.* Follow through and do what you say you will do. Be realistic about your energy and time; do not offer to do what you are unable to do.

    - *Sincerely apologize when you have done something to hurt or offend.*

Activities for Caregivers

Care Partners Activity #1: Who are my care partners?

Care Partners Checklist

Caregivers usually have family and friends who share in the caring. With a cooperative team, caregiving becomes easier. The wider and more helpful your network, the more strength you will have for caring. But when a caregiver is alone or when relationships among caregivers break down, helping becomes difficult. Use this chart to assess your caregiving partnerships and to identify possible new partners in care.

Directions: Check the box that describes the quality of support you receive from each of these parties. Check the blue box on the left to identify possible new partners in care.

I get cooperative support and effective help from:	Never, OR Does not apply to me	Very Rarely	With some regularity	Very often	Constantly	Possible New Partners
1. My spouse	0	1	2	3	4	
2. My child/children	0	1	2	3	4	
3. My sibling(s)/ brother- or sister-in-law	0	1	2	3		
4, My parent(s)	0	1	2	3	4	
5. My aunt(s)/uncle(s)	0	1	2	3	4	
6. My niece(s)/ nephew(s)	0	1	2	3	4	
7. My cousin(s)	0	1	2	3	4	
8. My grandchild/ children	0	1	2	3	4	
9. My grandparent(s)	0	1	2	3	4	
10. My neighbor(s)	0	1	2	3	4	
11. My friend(s)	0	1	2	3	4	
12. Members of my faith community	0	1	2	3	4	

13. Members of my support group	0	1	2	3	4	
14. Members of my online community	0	1	2	3	4	
15. Paid professionals who help me or my loved one	0	1	2	3	4	
To tally your score, add the numbers selected in each column, and then add the numbers across this bottom row. **My total score is:**_____	___	___	___	___	___	

©Partners on the Path. 2022. www.PartnersonthePath.com

Care Partners Activity #1: Interpreting My Score

These items provide a **snapshot of your support network**, the help you have for being a caregiver.

Total scores of 0-29, as well as **a response of 0 or 1 to most items** suggest *minimal, intermittent or poor quality support.* This puts you at risk for feeling alone and overburdened, for becoming overly reliant on a few people, and for becoming ill or burning out.

Protect yourself by actively expanding the size of your network and quality of support you receive. Open up; share your needs and feelings on a deeper level. Reach out to new people. Join online or in-person support groups. Use suggestions in the **Care Partners** text to help cultivate your community of support.

Total scores of 30 and above, as well as <u>responses of 3 or 4</u> on many items, indicates a *large and strong network.* Continue linking to these people to retain your health, well-being and capacity to care.

The maximum **score of 60** is unlikely; most people find that some categories do not apply to them.

Care Partners Activity #2: Who can help me with caregiving?

<u>Action Plan for Getting Help</u>

<u>Directions</u>: Are you sometimes **T-I-R-E-D** from all you do as a caregiver? Caregiving is a big job that others can help you handle if you request and accept offers of help. Follow these steps to use this Action Plan for Getting Help:

1. Review the left column of each checklist: 1. Tasks—2. Information—3. Respite—4. Emotional Support—5. Decisions and check the area(s) where you'd really like some help.

2. Now think of who could assist you with these tasks you checked.

3. Finally, identify what next steps you'll take to get the help you need.

4. Return to this checklist in the future when you need relief, support or hands-on-help with caregiving responsibilities.

1. Tasks Checklist			
Tasks for which I need help:	√	*Who could assist with these tasks?*	*Next Steps I'll take to get help:*
Physical Care: Help to feed, bathe, dress, groom, or help to walk, get to bathroom; to perform medical/nursing tasks.			
Personal Affairs: Help to cook, clean, shop, launder clothes, run errands, do home repairs or help with relocation.			
Household Affairs: Help to manage medicine, finances, legal, insurance, care coordination or transportation.			
Emotional or Social Support: Help with behavior, moods, socializing or making decisions.			

Action Plan for Getting Help (*Continued*)

2. Information Checklist			
The type of information I need:	√	*Who could provide this information?*	*Next Steps I'll take to get help:*
Medical: Diagnosis/condition, treatment options, professional referrals, health care organizations, medication management, medical equipment			
Care Management: Community resources, national/state programs, professional care coordinators, online/technology resources, housing, senior driving advice			
Legal/Financial: Private and public insurance providers, eldercare attorneys, Veteran benefits			

3. Respite Checklist			
The kind of break I need:	√	*Who could help arrange this time rest?*	*Next Steps I'll take to get help:*
Time out: Less than 30 minutes on an specific day/evening			
Mini-break: Several hours on a given day/evening			
Short getaway: Leave my loved one for a day or weekend			
Vacation: Leave my loved one for a week or more			

Action Plan for Getting Help (*Continued*)

4. Emotional Support Checklist			
Difficult emotions I'm feeling:	√	*Who could offer emotional support?*	*Next Steps I'll take to get help:*
Unprepared: I am **responsible** for coordinating care or providing complex medical/nursing care, **yet have no medical training**.			
Unpredictable: I have **no control** over if or when medical **emergencies and crises** will occur.			
Unrealistic: I manage **caregiving on top of my other responsibilities** to work, family and home. My **"to-do" lists are too much to do**.			
Unsupported: I receive **inadequate help** from family, friends, health care, insurance or legal systems. It's **hard to get a break** from my responsibilities.			
Upset: I am grappling with **complicated emotions**, feelings of loss, anger, sadness, guilt, depression, or fear. I'm unhappy with the **"new normal"** that I'm forced to accept.			
Under-funded: Paying **"out-of-pocket" for caregiving expenses** (supplies, services, or travel) is hurting my finances.			

Action Plan for Getting Help (*Continued*)

5. Decision Checklist			
Decisions I need help with:	√	*Who could help with decision making?*	*Next Steps I'll take to get help:*
Workplace issues-How to handle: Overload of work & caregiving responsibilities; conflict-culture isn't caregiver-friendly; need change & need income			
Family or personal issues-How to handle: Unbalanced family involvement; conflict; different caregiving priorities; loneliness; need for self-care			
Health care or medical treatment issues-How to handle: Problems with physical or mental health; cost/time barriers to staying healthy			
Legal or financial issues-How to handle: Costs of caregiving supplies, services or travel; loss of income or savings; power-of-attorney			

Care Partners Activity #3: Guided Self-Reflection

<u>Getting Nourished by My Care Partners: Guided Self-Reflection</u>

Directions: Like a well-stocked refrigerator, the people around you are filled with energy to help and sustain you. Use the following questions to help you explore how care partners nourish you.

1. Openness to Receiving Support

<u>Name It</u>
- Do I **"open the door"** to support from others, or tend to handle caregiving concerns on my own?
- What positive benefits do I get from my usual approach?
- What are the costs associated with not opening the door to others' support?

2. Reliable Sources of Support

<u>Name It</u>
- Who are my **"dependable brands"**, those friends and family who are reliable, realistic and really helpful people?
- Have I told them lately how much their support means? Offering recognition and thanks costs nothing but is an invaluable gift to the receiver. It is a sure way to keep relationships open and strong.

3. Undependable, Unable or Unwilling Supporters

<u>Name It</u>
- When have I looked for "*milk in an egg carton*," seeking support from someone unable or unwilling to provide what I needed? What was the outcome: did I get the help I requested? How comfortable did it feel?
- If the situation did not work well, is there another source I could turn to if I need that type of help in the future?
- Are there **"empty pitchers,"** in my community of support, people who are tired, over-committed, or out of balance in their own lives? Are there other sources I can turn to instead of these people? How do I feel when an "empty pitcher" lets me down?

©Partners on the Path. 2022. www.PartnersonthePath.com

Helpful Resources

Aging Life Care Association: https://www.aginglifecare.org// links you to certified professionals, formerly known as geriatric care managers, who partner with families to help plan and coordinate an elderly loved one's care.

Capossela, Cappy and Warnock, Sheila. *Share the Care: How to Organize a Group to Care for Someone Who Is Seriously Ill.* Fireside. Second Edition, 2004. Find additional resources on their website: *Share the Care*: https://sharethecare.org/

Caring for the Caregiver: Cultivate Community https://www.youtube.com/watch?v=6yzOLfhY3M0&t=27s YouTube video of the author describing the importance of connecting with care partners,

Caregiver Concerns: I feel so alone https://www.youtube.com/watch?v=lLJSfUJdIcU YouTube video from the author suggesting how caregiver can reach out for helpful information and emotional support.

Eldercare Locator: https://eldercare.acl.gov/Public/Index.aspx connects older Americans and their caregivers with community-based service providers throughout the country, linking to Area Agencies on Aging and organizations that serve older adults and their caregivers. Call the Eldercare Locator toll-free at 1-800-677-1116.

Ianacare: https://www.ianacare.com/ equips family caregivers with practical tools and supportive communities, so no one goes through the caregiving journey alone. Download the free app on their website, the Apple or Google App Store.

Mace, Nancy and Rabins, Peter. *The 36-Hour Day: A Family Guide to Caring for People Who Have Alzheimer Disease and Other Dementias.* Johns Hopkins University Press. 2021.

Well Spouse Association: https://wellspouse.org/ is a national, non-profit membership organization which gives support to wives, husbands, and partners of the chronically ill and/or disabled.

....

"Condemn none: if you can stretch out a helping hand, do so. If you cannot, fold your hands, bless your brothers, and let them go their own way."
Swami Vivekananda
Indian leader and Hindu teacher

"A small body of determined spirits fired by an unquenchable faith in their mission can alter the face of history."
Mohandas Gandhi
Indian leader and advocate of non-violent protest

"If we have no peace, it is because we have forgotten that we belong to each other."
Mother Theresa
Roman Catholic nun and humanitarian

....

CHAPTER 11

Resilience: Strength and Stamina to Cope with Adversity

Caregivers' Stories

Imagine the challenges faced by these caregivers.

- A young couple deeply grieves when learning that their newborn's Tay–Sachs disease that has no treatment or cure, and a life-expectancy of four years.

- A veteran's wife struggles to cope with her wounded warrior's traumatic brain injury and PTSD.

- A middle-aged woman tries to balance the needs of her aging parents with those of her growing family and her challenging work responsibilities.

- An elderly couple does what they can for each other; his Parkinson's and her pancreatic cancer are both advancing.

People of all ages and in an endless variety of situations care for loved ones and often wonder how they will manage. Fear, uncertainty, grief and exhaustion can be overwhelming. Though overwhelming, the challenges must be faced. Resilience gives caregivers strength and stamina to cope with adversity. How about you? If you are sad, stressed or stretched by the demands of caregiving, focus on building your resilience.

WHAT is resilience? WHY is it important for family caregivers?

Resilience is your *ability to withstand, recover, and sometimes grow when faced with adversity*; it is an *active process of enduring and successfully coping*. Resilience is *bouncing back after a crisis*. It's also *bouncing forward to adjust to a "new normal."*

This capacity to adapt and cope with adversity is present to varying degrees in every person, no matter how tumultuous external events or inner feelings may be. Fortunately, with attention and practice resilience can be strengthened. Resilience creates stamina and strength, expands capability and reduces vulnerability to stress. *Building resilience helps sustain caregiver health, well-being and capacity to care.*

HOW do resilient people handle adversity?

In *Resilience*, Steven Southwick and Dennis Charney (2018) outline *ten ways that resilient people tend to cope with stress. The good news is that these can be learned and developed.*

1. **Realistic Optimism:** Viewing life in a hopeful, confident way. Anticipating a bright future. Believing that good things are coming and hard work will yield success. *Realistic optimism is the foundation of resilience, and fuels each of the following resilience factors.*

2. **Social Support**: Connecting with other people by *seeking out and accepting help* that is offered, and also by giving help to those in need.

3. **Facing Fear:** Using thoughts and behaviors to triumph over fear. Acting in spite of fear to accomplish goals and become stronger.

4. **Religion and Spirituality:** Turning to God, or a Higher Power. Engaging in formal religious services or private spiritual practices. Finding inspiration in nature or the arts.

5. **Meaning, Purpose and Growth:** Finding strength and courage by pursuing an inspiring goal. Using adversity as a catalyst for growth. Actively serving a purpose that is greater than self-interest. Transcending traumatic experiences by helping others who have been traumatized. Choosing to be a victor, rather than a victim.

6. **Moral Compass/Altruism:** Engaging in right actions and avoiding doing wrong. Thinking of and serving others.

7. **Role models**: Imitating people who demonstrate positive ways of handling adversity. Identifying real people, living or dead; fictional characters, famous individuals or historic figures. Replicating small aspects of their behavior that have led to positive, desired outcomes.

8. **Training:** Improving physical health and preventing or diminishing the effects of chronic illnesses by keeping the body fit. Mastering physical challenges to also improve mental health and emotional regulation.

9. **Brain fitness:** Focusing thoughts, and challenging the mind so the intellect is sharp and continues to grow. Regulating emotions to eliminate feelings that undermine effective coping.

10. **Flexibility:** Employing a variety of mental and emotional strategies to handle adversity; accept what can't be changed; learn from failure; transform negative energy into positive energy; and find opportunity and meaning in adversity.

Source: Southwick, Steven and Charney, Dennis. *Resilience: The Science of Mastering Life's Greatest Challenges, 2nd Edition.* New York, Cambridge University Press. 2018.

HOW can I become more resilient?

Start by following Southwick and Charney's (2018) research findings and *work on building realistic optimism*. Listen to your thoughts; they create your reality. As soon as a negative thought comes, replace it with a positive one. When something positive happens, stop to acknowledge and appreciate the good. The more you challenge negative thinking and reinforce positive aspects of life, the more optimistic and resilient you will become.

Also, *review the ten resilience factors listed above; recall past difficulties and how you overcame them.* What did you do then when you bounced back, or coped well? These thoughts, choices or behaviors are examples of your approach to living with resilience. It would be helpful to *do something similar whenever you are faced with caregiving challenges.*

More Strategies on HOW to Build Resilience

Based on extensive research, the US military has developed a model for promoting resilience among their troops. The eight categories of resilience building strategies provide wise guidance for the general population, as well.

Review these additional eight strategies. To help you develop a resilience-building action plan, go to Resilience Activity #2 on page 153 of this chapter and use *Resilience Activity #2: What will I do to build my resilience?* Choose actions that work best for you. *Whatever you do to boost your resilience will be good for both you and for those in your care.*

Physical Strategies: Choose wisely to protect your fitness and health

Research shows that some simple physical strategies can successfully build resilience and preserve good health. Make these four items priorities in your life:

1. **Adequate Sleep:** *Sleep is not a waste of time or a luxury. Sleep is a productive time when your body and brain rejuvenate.* Sleep strengthens your immune system and balances out moods. It improves your memory, and helps you to focus, think and learn. Sleep deprivation increases stress and the risk of accidents; it can lead to high blood pressure, heart attack, stroke, obesity or depression. Most adults need 7-8 hours of sleep each night.

2. **Regular Movement:** *Physical activity boosts physical and mental health, improves sleep, reduces stress, increase alertness, and raises energy.* Combined with healthy eating, it can help prevent a host of chronic diseases. Guidelines suggest https://www.cdc.gov/physicalactivity/ that you should be active 30 minutes a day, 5 days a week.

   You don't need to go to a gym; any movement counts. Choose something you like, such as: walking, gardening, bowling, dancing, biking, or yoga. Any activity is better than none, so limit "screen time" and set goals to increase activity. Happily, if you are not currently fit you may see greater benefits from physical activity than those who are already fit.

3. **Good Grooming:** Cleanliness costs nothing more than the price of soap and toothpaste. Dressing well needn't be expensive, either. But personal grooming: cleaning your skin and clothes, using a lotion or attractive scent, keeping hair clean and neatly combed, and keeping clothes in good repair all help you to look and feel good. *Good grooming and healthy personal habits help you ward off illnesses, help you feel good about yourself, and attract others to you.*

4. **Avoiding harm:** *Stay safe by being careful with medications, alcohol and tobacco.* Use medications as prescribed and dispose of those that are outdated. Never share prescribed drugs with another person. If you have questions about prescriptions, ask your primary care provider or pharmacist. If you are taking a variety

of medications, be sure to share this list with your physician and pharmacist.

Drink alcohol in moderation or not at all. Guidelines on alcohol http://www.cdc.gov/alcohol/faqs.htm define moderate drinking as up to 2 drinks per day for men and 1 drink per day for women. It is not safe to drink and drive, or to drink when pregnant. Smoking or chewing tobacco is never safe.

Physical Strategies for Resilient Caregivers

None of these ideas are difficult, but choosing them can be. *Disciplined, healthy choices are wise; they recognize that physical self-care isn't a nicety, it's a necessity.* As a caregiver, protecting your physical fitness and health benefits you and those in your care. If your energy drains away and your body breaks down, caregiving tasks that were once manageable will become difficult or impossible to do. Make healthy choices to boost your resilience and preserve your capacity to care.

Nutritional Strategies: Select healthy foods and eating behaviors

How Good Nutrition Helps Caregivers

Nutritious eating promotes good health, building strength and stamina needed for providing care. It *helps decrease a caregiver's risk for developing minor ailments or more serious chronic illnesses*. And good nutrition *strengthens the immune system's ability fight illnesses* that do arise.

Poor nutrition leads to fatigue and illness, increasing the risk for serious health problems. It leads to *longer recovery times, increased risk of infections and greater risk of falls*. Choosing nutritious food is one of the most powerful things a caregiver can do to stay healthy, build resilience and continue caring. A resilient caregiver eats a healthy diet. (For more: http://www.weightandwellness.com/resources/articles-and-videos/

articles-about-other-health-conditions/nutrition-the-foundation-of-sel f-care-for-caregivers/)

Nutritional Strategies that Work

Research shows that good nutrition for caregivers is based on healthful food choices and eating behaviors. Take these three steps toward better nutrition:

1. **Eat a Balanced Diet:** A well balanced diet provides the energy and nutrients your body needs to function, remain healthy, and grow. Guidelines on https://www.choosemyplate.gov emphasize:

    -   Choosing colorful fruits and vegetables, whole grains, lean fish and poultry, low-fat dairy products

    -   Limiting red meat, sugar, salt or saturated fats like butter

    -   Controlling portion size, sugary drinks, and the quantity of snacks or comfort foods.

    The Mayo Clinic adds that drinking at least eight 8-ounce glasses of fluid a day is another important part of a healthy diet. https://www.mayoclinic.org/healthy-lifestyle/nutrition-and-healthy-eating/in-depth/water/art-20044256

    In The National Institutes of Health's e-book, *What's on Your Plate: Smart Food Choices for Healthy Aging* https://order.nia. nih.gov/sites/default/files/2022-12/whats-on-your-plate-nia. pdf you can learn all the basics about food types, recommended daily calories, portion size, sample menus, and overcoming roadblocks to healthy eating.

2. **Select Healthy Snacks:** Though often discouraged, eating between meals can actually be good for holding off hunger and keeping energy high. The trick is to choose wisely and eat

in moderation. Look for foods that are proteins, fresh fruits or vegetables, whole grains or low-fat dairy, rather than simple starches, refined sugars or processed foods. The American Heart Association recommends selecting nutrient-rich foods like these:

Crunchy

- Apples and Breadsticks
- Carrot and celery sticks
- Green pepper sticks
- Zucchini circles
- Radishes
- Broccoli spears
- Cauliflower
- Unsalted rice cakes

Munchy

- Unsalted sunflower seeds
- Whole-grain breads or toast
- Cherry or grape tomatoes
- Low-fat or fat-free cheese
- Plain, low-fat or fat-free yogurt
- Bagels
- Unsalted almonds, walnuts and other nuts

Thirst Quenchers

- Fat-free milk
- Unsweetened juices
- Low-sodium tomato or mixed vegetable juice
- Water

Sweet

- Unsweetened canned fruit
- Thin slice of angel food cake
- Baked apple
- Raisins
- Dried fruit gelatin gems
- Frozen bananas
- Frozen grapes
- Fresh fruit
- Low-fat unsweetened fruit yogurt

When snacking, limit calorie intake; it's a snack, not another meal! For some ideas on low-cal choices, check out these links:

https://www.webmd.com/diet/ss/slideshow-100-calorie-snacks

https://www.healthline.com/nutrition/29-healthy-snacks-for-weight-loss#TOC_TITLE_HDR_3

3. **Overcome Barriers to Healthy Eating:** At some time all of us make unwise eating choices. Which of these barriers apply to you?

- <u>Overindulging</u>: Processed foods, sweets, salty snacks, high fat foods; frequent fast-food meals or restaurant meals

- <u>Under-selecting</u>: Too few fresh vegetables, fruits, whole grains, lean protein, low-fat dairy, not drinking enough water, skipping meals

- <u>Lack of self-control</u>: Binge eating, overeating to point of being stuffed, frequent snacking

- <u>Emotional eating</u>: When anxious, depressed, lonely, angry, frustrated or bored

- <u>Not preparing healthy food</u>: No time, too tired, too busy, too expensive, don't know how, family/friends won't eat healthy food if I prepare it

Replacing these unwise choices and behaviors with more nutritious ones will improve your health, increase your resilience and sustain your energy for caregiving. Check-out these links for some ways to overcome your barriers to healthy eating:

- https://food-guide.canada.ca/en/tips-for-healthy-eating/

- https://www.psycom.net/stop-emotional-eating

Healthy Nutrition for Resilient Caregivers

None of these ideas are difficult, but choosing them can be. Disciplined, healthy eating patterns are an important way to build your strength and stamina. Protecting your wellbeing benefits both you and those in your care. Use these nutritional strategies to boost your resilience and preserve your capacity to care.

Medical Strategies: Take practical steps to protect your health

Practical Ways to Protect Your Health

Common sense recognizes that healthy bodies are better able to function and handle adversity. Many caregivers encourage loved ones to manage their health by visiting the doctor, scheduling preventive screenings, or monitoring medications. But *caregivers often neglect their own health*. Don't put your health at risk. Take these practical steps to protect your health.

1. **Access quality health care**

   This is the critical first step in protecting your health. Healthcare insurance provides access to care and it comes through employer-provided or government plans: Medicare, Medicaid, the Children's Health Insurance Program or Veterans Administration benefits. Without some form of insurance, preventive screenings and health care services are out of reach for most people.

   - For information about applying for Medicare, visit: http://www.ssa.gov/retire2/justmedicare.htm

   - Enrollment for Medicare can be done online: https://www.ssa.gov/medicare/sign-up

   - For Medicaid or the Children's Health Insurance Program (CHIP), apply directly to these agencies in your state. If you qualify, coverage can begin immediately.

   - If you qualify for Veterans' health benefits, contact the US Department of Veterans Affairs https://www.va.gov/

health-care/about-va-health-benefits/ The simplest way to apply is by submitting an online application at: https://www.va.gov/health-care/how-to-apply/

- The Patient Protection and Affordable Care Act (ACA) has made it possible for millions of Americans without access to employer-based or other government plans, to obtain affordable health insurance. For information, visit: https://www.healthcare.gov/get-coverage/

To help people with new coverage, the Federal government's Centers for Medicare and Medicaid Services (CMS) has created From Coverage to Care. The cornerstone of this initiative is an eight-step roadmap intended to guide the newly insured through the process of getting health care. The steps include:

Step 1: Put your health first
Step 2: Understand your health coverage
Step 3: Know where to go for care
Step 4: Pick a provider
Step 5: Make an appointment
Step 6: Be prepared for your visit
Step 7: Decide if the provider is right for you
Step 8: Next steps after your appointment

Find information about available health coverage and connect to the primary care and the preventive services that are right for you at: https://www.cms.gov/priorities/health-equity/c2c For information in any one of 18 different languages: https://www.cms.gov/priorities/health-equity/minority-health/resource-center/language

2. **Prevent health problems**

Protect your health with preventive care and screenings. These decrease the risk of serious illnesses and increase the likelihood of finding conditions early, when they are most manageable.

Every year, millions of Americans die of preventable deaths. Leading causes of death include: chronic diseases like diabetes, cardiovascular and respiratory illnesses; unintentional injuries and certain infections. *Prevent health problems with these simple, yet effective lifestyle choices*:

- Eat a balanced diet
- Maintain a healthy weight
- Exercise regularly
- Do not smoke or use other tobacco products
- Limit intake of alcohol
- Wash your hands
- Wear seatbelts each time you ride in a vehicle
- Get recommended immunizations

In addition to healthy lifestyle choices, preventive health care is a critically important way of maintaining your resilience and capacity to care. *Regularly visit a primary care provider to check for potential problems with screenings* that include:

- Dental, vision and hearing tests
- Cancer checks: Skin, colorectal, breast, cervical, testicular and prostate cancer
- Obesity, blood pressure, cholesterol, diabetes, infectious diseases screens
- For women, bone density tests

View health maintenance guidelines for adults: https://my.clevelandclinic.org/-/scassets/files/org/patients-visitors/information/health-maintenance-guidelines-for-adults.pdf?la=en

3. **Manage health problems**

Chronic conditions, physical injuries and related pain deplete energy and make it harder to care for others. *Chronic conditions are long-lasting, and can be controlled but not cured.* Examples include:

- Asthma
- Back and neck pain
- Diabetes
- Heart disease and high blood pressure
- Obesity
- Mental health problems
- Substance abuse

Although chronic conditions are among the most common and costly health problems, they are also among the most preventable and most can be effectively controlled. *When untreated or poorly managed, chronic conditions, pain, or injuries limit stamina and physical capabilities. They can lead to depression, and disrupt family and work-life.* Proper diagnosis, treatment, physical rehab and supportive therapies are crucial. Be proactive about managing your health. For additional information: https://www.webmd. com/depression/chronic-illnesses-depression

Medical Strategies for Resilient Caregivers

Acknowledging the importance of your own health isn't difficult, but it's often difficult finding time for self-care. *Remember that you can't help if you can't function. Don't let sickness or injury keep you from providing the care you want to give.* Use these medical strategies to protect your health and preserve your capacity to care.

Environmental Strategies: Draw energy from your home, imagination, and nature

How Your Environment Can Build Resilience

Connecting with the natural world and finding sanctuary in our home environment are proven sources of resilient energy. Hundreds of studies confirm that direct contact with nature reduces stress. It also promotes mental health and spiritual development; strengthens self-confidence and self-discipline; and improves connection to others in the community. Even indirect contact -- viewing nature through a window or having indoor plants -- has been shown to speed recovery and improve memory, concentration, satisfaction and work performance.

Source: http://ellisonchair.tamu.edu/health-and-well-being-benefit s-of-plants/#.VOYHHvnF9PM

In *Bouncing Back* (2013), author Linda Graham describes the value of creating a place of refuge, which she defines as a "safe, supportive place to be when we are fragile or confused, a safe place to cry or rant as long as we need to, or somewhere to wait patiently until a course of action begins to emerge from the chaos…In this refuge, we replenish ourselves. We help our nervous systems return to, or remain in, the state of physiological calm and equanimity called the 'window of tolerance'." This place of refuge can be real, in our homes, or it can be envisioned in our minds. Evoking a safe haven in the imagination can feel as real to the brain as a real, physical place.

Connecting with a Nurturing Environment

Use these three strategies when your caregiving journey is difficult. They will help you tap into refreshing energy that is all around you.

1. **Get close to nature.**

   Study nature, love nature, stay close to nature. It will never fail you. Frank Lloyd Wright

There are countless ways to connect with the healing, stress-reducing power of nature. The simplest way to recharge is to step outside your door and inhale deeply. Feel the sun's warmth, the cool raindrops, or frigid blast of falling snow the on your skin. Look up into the dark night sky; wonder at the moon and stars, or the dense covering of clouds. Listen for birds singing or the wind rustling the leaves. Drink it in and be grateful for whatever nature has in store for you at the moment.

With more time, go beyond your doorstep, alone or with others. Go to the nearest lake, river or seashore; take a picnic lunch or go fishing. Hike in the hills or just stroll around your neighborhood. Play at the park with a little child. Walk barefoot in the grass or sand; wade in a puddle. Dig in the dirt. Nibble a freshly-picked herb from the garden. Stop and smell the roses. Let all five senses drink in the beauty, and be calmed by the grandeur and order all around. Spend time outside; it isn't expensive but it's a priceless way to give your body and mind a rest.

For more ideas: http://www.enkicharity.com/fun-things-to-do-outside.html

Finally, find the grace to flow with peaks and valleys of your life by reflecting on the cycles of nature. The cold of winter gives way to small buds of spring. The full-flower of summer can't last forever; autumn's decline has a peace and beauty all its own. As caregivers, it's good to be reminded that, no matter how difficult the winter, spring always comes.

2. **Make your house a haven.**

Home is where one starts from. T. S. Eliot

Our energy for meeting life's challenges can be restored by returning to a home that nurtures us. To make your house such a restorative place, first *assure that it is a safe environment*. Take steps to prevent accidents or injuries.

- The home safety checklist from AARP is a helpful guide. https://createthegood.aarp.org/content/dam/aarp/ctg/pdf/guides/home-safety-individual.pdf

- The American Academy of Orthopaedic Surgeons suggestion ways to prevent falls, a major cause of serious injury to people of all ages, especially for the elderly. http://orthoinfo.aaos.org/topic.cfm?topic=A00123

- Prepare for emergencies by following this Red Cross Plan. http://www.redcross.org/prepare/location/home-family

- Implement these affordable ways to make your home safer and healthier. https://www.webmd.com/a-to-z-guides/features/affordable-ways-to-make-home-safer

- Organize important papers so they're easily accessible when you need them. https://www.caregiver.org/uploads/2022/02/ENGLISH_find_important_papers_form-211210.pdf

After addressing safety, focus on creating comfort. Home won't feel like a refuge if the environment is unsettled. What are irritants that bother you, things like noise, air quality, heat, cold, drafts or clutter? Identify what could reduce these stressors and help make your home a haven that feels good to you. Then take steps to bring these qualities into your home: clean up a messy room; organize your desk, a drawer or your files; de-clutter the kitchen counter; bring in flowers or a house plant; turn down bright lights; play soothing music. Do whatever will help settle your jangled nerves or shift your energy level. Anything that promotes beauty, calm, cleanliness or order can feed you with resilient energy, a great help when caregiving is challenging.

3. **Go to a safe place in your mind.**

Meditation can help us embrace our worries, our fear, our anger; and that is very healing. We let our own natural capacity of healing do the work. Thich Nhat Hanh

Guided imagery is a therapeutic technique. You can use it to create calm in your internal environment. *Safe Place Guided Imagery is a popular meditation you can use to relax* your nervous system and emotions, shift from negative to more positive thinking and regain a sense of balance and control. Use this link to try visiting your safe place: https://www.youtube.com/watch?v=pPBxNLpOLNU

When caregiving is painful or overwhelming, use this practice to create inner calm. Download this Safe Place Guided Imagery to help you adopt this as one of your resilience-building strategies. http://envisionintegrativetherapies.com/PDF/SAFE%20PLACE%20GUIDED%20IMAGERY.pdf

Environmental Strategies for Resilient Caregivers

Going to a safe haven in your home, your heart or in the natural world isn't difficult, but getting there can be. Don't let commitments, concerns or clutter block your way to a place of peace. Whatever you do to connect with a safe, calm environment will be good for both you and those in your care.

Psychological Strategies: Use your mind and mindfulness practices

Use Your Mind to Build Resilience

Throughout history, wisdom writers have advised us to respect the power of the mind.

- *Ideas are the source of all things. ~Plato*
- *We are what we think; all that we are arises in our thoughts. With our thoughts we make the world.~ Buddha*
- *Man often becomes what he believes himself to be. ~Mahatma Gandhi*
- *Change your thoughts and you change your world. ~Norman Vincent Peale*

21ˢᵗ century research bears out the wisdom of the ages. Boost your resilience with these two mental practices.

1. **Realistic Optimism**

   If you paint in your mind a picture of bright and happy expectations, you put yourself into a condition conducive to your goal. ~Norman Vincent Peale

   Optimism and pessimism are choices about how to look at the world, powerful thought patterns that can be changed with practice. Where *pessimists* are stopped by adverse conditions, *unrealistic optimists* are Pollyanna's who unwisely plunge ahead, ignoring real needs or threats. Neither of these promote resilience.

   Instead, choose *realistic optimism*, a lens that acknowledges reality and promotes clear thinking. Strongly related to resilience, realistic optimism promotes good health, successful relationships and strength to handle adversity.

   Practice these thought patterns to think like a realistic optimist:

- **Count your blessings**: Recognize all the good in your life and expect more to come. View negative experiences as isolated events or flukes that are unlikely to be repeated.

- **Take credit:** See that your efforts have brought good into your life. Recognize how actions of others, or factors beyond your control have contributed to your difficulties.

- **Expect more good:** Envision positive events continuing or being repeated in the future. Dismiss negative ones as unlikely to happen again.

- **Emphasize the positive:** No matter what the facts of the situation, think positive thoughts, but don't deny reality.

For more:

- On optimism and your health: https://www.health.harvard.edu/heart-health/optimism-and-your-health

- On ways to improve your optimism: https://positivepsychology.com/optimism-tools-exercises-examples/

2. Positive Self-Talk

When the mind is thinking it is talking to itself. ~Plato

"Self-talk" is the silent conversation that runs in the back of your mind about yourself and the world around you. Whether conscious or unconscious, this commentary powerfully shapes your feelings, energy and resilience. When exhausted, depressed or out of control, thoughts often turn negative. In times like these, you can build resilience by consciously using these positive self-talk practices.

- **Refocus attention**: When your mind is distracted, anxious, uncertain, or preoccupied with something, consciously switch to positive self-talk. *Change your focus to any other thought.* When anxiously awaiting results of surgery read a good book, or talk with someone about something other you're your worries. The mind can't think two thoughts at the same time.

- **Think positive thoughts**: When your thoughts become grouchy, defeatist, or negative, replace them with positive thoughts. Exchange, "This is awful! I can't handle this anymore!" with positive self-talk, "This may not be good but I'll manage." *Whatever you do to eliminate negative thoughts can help reduce anxiety and depression.*

- **Savor**: When something positive happens, stop and savor it, especially when you're feeling negative. Think, "Despite the dementia, we enjoyed the beautiful sunshine and a wonderful walk today." Reinforce a positive experience by thinking more encouraging thoughts. Recognize, "I did so well juggling my work and caregiving today; I know I'll be able to do it again." *Stop to appreciate and be grateful for goodness.*

For more:

- On self-talk: https://positivepsychology.com/positive-self-talk/

- On how to *Learn to Think Like an Optimist*: https://www.youtube.com/watch?v=MpedWDuwGzI

Use Mindfulness Practices to Build Resilience

Mindfulness involves *being attentive to present thoughts, feelings, physical sensations and surroundings; accepting these without judgment and without letting thoughts anxiously focus on past or future concerns.* Mindful breathing and mindfulness meditation are two key methods for reducing anxiety and creating inner calm.

1. **Mindful Breathing:** You breathe continuously, usually without awareness. Practice observing your breath without reacting; simply attend to it and feel it without attempting to change it. By intentionally focusing on your breath you can ground yourself in the present moment.

   Deep breathing lowers your heart rate, anxiety and muscle tension. It is the easiest way to elicit the relaxation response. In moments of high stress, pay attention to your breathing; breathe slowly and deeply from your abdomen. For the on-going stress of caregiving, make it a practice to breathe slowly and deeply for at least three minutes every day.

   Try this deep breathing activity to calm yourself and reenergize. Despite the busyness of daily schedules, or perhaps because of it, taking time for silence is critical to a caregiver's well-being. You don't need hours; even a few minutes will help. Follow these steps:

   1. *Go to a quiet space where you will not be interrupted.* Turn off the radio, television, computer, beeper and phone. Settle into a comfortable chair or sofa. Place your feet on the ground or put your feet up, if you like. Close your eyes.

   2. *Take in a deep breath from way down in your belly; fill your lungs and slowly exhale.* Slowly repeat this several times and feel yourself start to relax. Continue sitting quietly, breathing deeply, rhythmically, slowly. Clear your mind of all thoughts by focusing on inhaling and exhaling. Breathe in peace and calm. Breathe out tension and pain.

   3. *Gently refocus on inhaling and exhaling when your mind starts wandering* and thinking of other things, as it certainly will. Maintain a passive attitude; don't judge or get upset

about these thoughts. Simply notice them; picture them as balloons and let them float away. Refocus on breathing in peace and calm; breathing out tension and pain.

4. *Start by spending three minutes a day on this deep breathing activity.* Work up to twenty minutes.

5. *When the time is up, gradually open your eyes and pay attention to the feeling of calm.* Savor this feeling.

There are many exercises for developing mindful breathing. Check this link for guidance from wellness expert, Dr. Andrew Weil: https://www.drweil.com/health-wellness/body-mind-spirit/stress-anxiety/breathing-three-exercises/

2. **Mindfulness Meditation:** Formal meditation practice is rooted in ancient Buddhism, and because of its holistic health benefits, has been adopted by western culture. Mindfulness meditation is practiced sitting upright on a chair with eyes closed, or cross-legged on a cushion. Attention is focused on breathing in and out, as described above in the breathing activity. Instead of the breath, a word or phrase may be chosen as a focal point, *e.g.* "God," "peace," or "I am loved."

Thoughts that arise are recognized in an accepting, non-judgmental way; then focus is returned to the breath, word or phrase. Those who practice meditation often start with a short periods of 10 minutes each day. With regular practice, time spent meditating is extended; it becomes easier to keep focused attention and to experience the calming benefits of meditation.

Psychology Today presents an overview of mindfulness meditation: http://www.psychologytoday.com/blog/the-courage-be-present/201001/how-practice-mindfulness-meditation

Try this video to experience a brief guided meditation: https://www.youtube.com/watch?v=dEzbdLn2bJc

Psychological Strategies for Resilient Caregivers

Using your mind and mindfulness practices aren't difficult, but choosing them can be. Uncertainty can get in the way of choosing unfamiliar mindfulness practices. Changing ingrained patterns can be very hard, especially when feeling worn down by the challenges of caregiving. Don't let hesitations, old habits or fatigue hinder you from experiencing the benefits of these resilience-building practices.

Social Strategies: Reach out and connect with others

Social Support Builds Resilience

Social support refers to providing informational, emotional, or tangible, "hands-on" help. Researchers have demonstrated that social support builds resilience when it helps people face difficult situations, or promotes the use of healthy behaviors.

In *Resilience,* Steven Southwick and Dennis Charney (2018) report on multiple studies that describe the benefits of strong, positive relationships. *Connecting with others relieves stress, improves physical health and prolongs life. Good support from others also enhances emotional well-being and protects against depression.*

Practical Ways to Connect and Build Resilience

Knowing the power of social support, try these strategies to reach out and connect with others.

1. **Connect to help and support**

   Ask for and be open to receiving help. Even if you dislike doing it, ask others to help with tasks, give advice, share contacts or simply listen. *Caregiving is too big a job to handle on your own.*

If you're overwhelmed, or simply very busy, reach out for help. Name your needs and people who might be willing to help. Check the **Action Plan for Getting Help** found in Care Partners Activity #2 of Chapter 10 on page 111: Care Partners. It will prepare you to respond when someone asks, "How can I help?"

And check-out these two great resources:

• **Lotsa Helping Hands** http://www.lotsahelpinghands.com/ is a free, online community that offers tools that help caregivers connect with volunteers who want to offer support. A Lotsa App can be downloaded from the App Store or Google Play Store.

• **Share the Care** http://sharethecare.org/ is a practical, step-by-step model for creating a "caregiving group" who will come together to support someone facing a health or aging crisis. Proven effective and available both online and as a paperback, these guidelines are easy to replicate and eliminate the need to reinvent the wheel.

2. **Connect to understanding and empathy**

Reach out when you're lonely or sad. Don't withdraw into your own world. Even if it's hard, connect to others via phone calls, texts, emails, Zoom chats, notes or friendly visits. Meet a friend for coffee or to take a walk together. *Even brief, informal exchanges with others can give you positive energy.*

When reaching out, stretch beyond your immediate circle of family and friends. Online caregiver organizations, condition-related organizations and faith communities are places where you can connect with people who understand and support caregivers.

Join a support group. If you have mixed feelings about joining, know that you're not alone! Noted psychologist, Barry Jacobs describes groups that work, and why some aren't so successful. But he is clear that, "all family caregivers can benefit from talking with others in similar situations."

There is a wealth of online support for caregivers. Google "support groups for caregivers" or follow these links:

- Alzheimer's Association: https://www.alz.org/events/event_search?etid=2&cid=0

- Family Caregiver Alliance: https://www.caregiver.org/connecting-caregivers/support-groups/

3. **Connect to hope and inspiration**

Resilient people gain strength and hope from imitating their role models (Southwick and Charney, 2018). Think of people who have successfully handled adversity, hardships and challenges. They may be real folks you know or who you've only heard about; people who are alive or dead; fictional characters from a movie or book; historic figures or famous people from any walk of life. Identify qualities or specific behaviors that helped them get through, or that yielded the outcome you desire. Then, *replicate that behavior.*

As an example, the story of how Vietnam POW's survived three years in solitary confinement may inspire you. It reveals the power of human connection and our capacity to survive adversity. In a YouTube video: https://www.youtube.com/watch?v=3zUImnnjCtI you'll see how their "tap code" connected POW's and sustained their lives. For the full story, read this book: *Tap Code: The Epic Survival Tale of a Vietnam POW and the Secret Code That Changed Everything.* Have confidence in your resilience. Remember that all things pass away…including difficult times! *Think of how the "tap code" helped the POW's. Imitate them by finding ways to communicate and connect with others.*

Social Strategies for Resilient Caregivers

Reaching out and connecting with others isn't complicated, but it can be difficult to do. Fatigue, depression, busy-ness, embarrassment and resentment are just a few things that block caregivers from connecting with others. Don't let barriers like these hinder you from receiving life-giving support.

Spiritual Strategies: Reflect, connect, and give thanks

Spiritual Beliefs and Practices Build Resilience

Spirituality is an aspect of every human life. Deeply held beliefs that guide and give meaning act as lenses through which we see the world, and as ethical guides for how we act in the world. Spirituality can be experienced through both religious and secular practices. *Religious practices* include prayer, worship, reading scripture or religious meditation. *Secular practices* include appreciating nature and the arts; participating in yoga or volunteer work.

Spiritual Resources for Caregivers

When your caregiving journey is difficult, use spiritual resources like these to build inner strength and stamina.

- **Reflection:** *Consider the purpose and value of all you do as a caregiver.* Spend quiet time alone. Capture your thoughts and feelings by journaling. Talk with a counselor or clergy person, a friend or family member who you trust.

  Noted 20ᵗʰ Century spiritual writer, Henri Nouwen, has written *A Spirituality of Caregiving: Reflections on the joys and anguish of caregiving.* Nouwen shares insights on what it means to be a caregiver and to be cared for.

- **Connection:** *Commune with nature* to be reminded of a Higher Power that created and sustains the universe, throughout all time and in all circumstances. Spend time at a park, near the ocean or a lake, in the forest, on a hillside or mountain. Look and listen; absorb the power and beauty. Find rest and renewal in nature.

  Connect with God through prayer, worship, scriptures or meditation. Through this connection, you can feel the presence of a Higher Power upholding you during times of trial. If you've never actively prayed, or if it's been a long time, give it a try and see how it feels. An interesting blog on this topic can be found at: https://youragingparent.com/

- **Gratitude:** *Giving thanks is the root of peace and joy.* Regularly savor good and enjoyable aspects of your life; they're not owed to you, but are gifts. Read this post to learn more about gratitude and why it's so important: https://www.psychologytoday.com/us/basics/gratitude

  Deepen your gratitude by taking time at the start or end of each day to give thanks for people and things that bless your life. Or set the alarm on your smart phone to ring each day; when you hear it, recall three things for which you give thanks.

  In a Daily Gratitude Journal write a list of things you're grateful for each day. Write a letter of gratitude to someone who has especially touched your life and tell them what their care has meant to you. Sign-up to receive daily quotes about gratitude from www.gratefulness.org

Spiritual Practices for Resilient Caregivers

Reflection, connection and gratitude aren't difficult to do, but task-driven busy-ness can get in the way of these practices. *Don't let the world's agenda steal your time for spiritual sustenance.* Because this is a personal journey, no one spiritual resource works for everyone. Select practices that work well for you. Add them to other physical, mental and social strategies you use to build resilience.

Family Strategies: Cultivate the qualities of resilient families

Family resilience: Why it matters

While some families are shattered by crises or chronic stress, others pull together and are strengthened. What distinguishes one from the other is family resilience. Building your family's resilience creates stamina, strength and the capacity to cope. It decreases vulnerability to stress; helps you solve problems, sustains your health, well-being and capacity to care.

Resilience is present to varying degrees in both individuals and families. Fortunately, with attention and practice family resilience can be strengthened.

How Resilient Families Handle Adversity

Dr. Froma Walsh tells us there are nine ways that resilient families handle adversity. They:

1. **Think optimistically:** Holding a positive, rather than pessimistic outlook on life; recognizing one another's strengths; offering words of encouragement; accepting what's beyond control or can't be changed.

2. **Find meaning in adversity:** Labeling crises as manageable and shared challenges; accepting difficult feelings as human and understandable under the circumstances; believing in the family's ability to learn, grow and move beyond this difficult experience.

3. **Cultivate spirituality**: Holding beliefs and values that offer meaning, purpose and connection; finding strength and comfort in cultural or religious traditions; seeking spiritual inspiration in nature, the arts, service to others, and faith in a higher power.

4. **Exhibit flexibility:** Adapting to change; adjusting family roles and rules while maintaining rituals and traditions that provide stability; providing for children strong, yet nurturing guidance and protection; demonstrating mutual respect in the marital relationship.

5. **Connect and collaborate:** Pulling together as a team during times of crisis; supporting each other while respecting individual needs, differences and boundaries.

6. **Tap their resources:** Reaching-out for help when problems can't be solved on their own; getting assistance from extended family, friends, neighbors, community agencies and/or counseling.

7. **Openly share emotions:** Accepting and encouraging a wide range of emotional expression (joy, sadness, fear, silliness, etc.) in adults and children; taking individual responsibility for one's own feelings and accepting others who have different feelings; valuing positive interactions and humor, even during difficult circumstances.

8. **Clearly communicate:** Communicating in understandable, consistent and honest ways; saying what they mean and meaning what they say, so as to avoid sending vague, confusing or mixed messages.

9. **Collaborate on problem solving:** Working together to understand problems and ways to solve them; making decisions together; allowing open sharing of disagreements; resolving disagreements through negotiation, compromise and give-and-take; repairing hurts and misunderstandings that go along with

conflicts; proactively solving current problems so as to prevent future ones; learning from mistakes.

Cultivating you family's resilience

You can build your family's resilience by cultivating any of the qualities Walsh identified in her book, *Strengthening Family Resilience (2006)*. While building family resilience isn't complicated, it can seem too difficult to do, especially when you're overloaded with responsibilities or overwhelmed with stress. These tips can help.

- **Inform**: Share this list with other family members and the benefits of family resilience. Discuss which of these they'd be willing to work on.

- **Simplify**: Start by strengthening just one of these nine qualities. Pick one that would most easily lead to positive outcomes and a sense of success.

- **Brainstorm**: Ask, "What can we do to strengthen this quality?" Agree on a "to-do" list. Review materials on resilience that are found elsewhere in this book.

- **Collaborate**: Engage everyone in some way; those of all ages can contribute. Working together can create positive energy, much needed by caregiving families.

- **Celebrate**: Recognize accomplishments. Praise positive contributions. Rejoice over successes.

- **Persevere**: Don't be discouraged if you don't feel immediate positive results. Overtime, the investment in building family strength pays off.

- **Expand**: Build on your success. Gain more positive energy by nurturing the development of additional resilience factors.

Because your family and your caregiving experience are unique, *no one set of recommendations will work for everyone. Cultivate those qualities that will nurture your family.* Whatever you do to foster healthy, resilient relationships will be good for all of you.

Activities for Caregivers

Resilience Activity #1: How resilient am I?

<u>Resilience Project Self-Evaluation</u>

<u>Directions</u>: Evaluate your level of resilience using specific numbers or indicators of your general feeling about each statement. Please answer all items!

<u>For Numerical Ranking</u>: Next to each statement you will see a scale from 0 to 10. 0 stands for "does not apply to me at all" and 10 stands for "I fully agree." Choose the number that applies to you. You will get 0-30 points for each of the seven categories of questions.

PERCEPTION											Section Score:
1. I believe that my life is meaningful and worth living.	0	1	2	3	4	5	6	7	8	9	10
2. I notice new and positive things more often than negative and well-known things.	0	1	2	3	4	5	6	7	8	9	10
3. I am aware of my feelings without allowing them to control me.	0	1	2	3	4	5	6	7	8	9	10
GETTING A GRIP OF ONE'S LIFE											Section Score:
4. I believe that I can influence my life situation and am not a victim of the circumstances.	0	1	2	3	4	5	6	7	8	9	10
5. I approach things (pleasant and unpleasant) and take action.	0	1	2	3	4	5	6	7	8	9	10
6. I set clear priorities for my life.	0	1	2	3	4	5	6	7	8	9	10

FORMING RELATIONSHIPS Section Score:

7. I have at least one person in my life with whom I can share everything – the good & the bad.	0	1	2	3	4	5	6	7	8	9	10
8. I make time for the people that are important to me.	0	1	2	3	4	5	6	7	8	9	10
9. I have faith in others and I can rely on their support when I need it.	0	1	2	3	4	5	6	7	8	9	10

ACCEPTANCE & OPTIMISTIC THINKING (*CONFIDENCE IN FUTURE*) Section Score:

10. I look forward to a bright future and know I can handle difficulties.	0	1	2	3	4	5	6	7	8	9	10
11. I evaluate my experiences and learn from mistakes as well as successes.	0	1	2	3	4	5	6	7	8	9	10
12. I adapt flexibly to change and easily accept the unchangeable.	0	1	2	3	4	5	6	7	8	9	10

ORIENTATION ON SOLUTIONS AND AIMS Section Score:

13. I prefer finding solutions to searching for mistakes and someone to blame.	0	1	2	3	4	5	6	7	8	9	10
14. I am aware of my visions and am prepared to fulfill my own wishes.	0	1	2	3	4	5	6	7	8	9	10
15. I have goals for my life and they are consistent with my values.	0	1	2	3	4	5	6	7	8	9	10

HEALTHY LIFESTYLE											Section Score:
16. I am important to myself and I take good care of myself.	0	1	2	3	4	5	6	7	8	9	10
17. I am in touch with my body and feel what's good for me and what's not.	0	1	2	3	4	5	6	7	8	9	10
18. In a difficult situation, I put my own health before the expectations of others.	0	1	2	3	4	5	6	7	8	9	10

SELF-EFFICACY											Section Score:
19. I know what I am capable of and am confident in myself.	0	1	2	3	4	5	6	7	8	9	10
20. I can rely on my own abilities and resources in difficult times.	0	1	2	3	4	5	6	7	8	9	10
21. I believe in myself.	0	1	2	3	4	5	6	7	8	9	10

Scoring: Add-up the numbers you circled. **To interpret your score, see the Scoring Guide.**   My score is: _____

Source: Resilience Project (open access)
http://www.resilience-project.eu/uploads/media/self_evaluation_en.pdf

Resilience Project Self-Evaluation: Scoring Guide

Complete the evaluation by looking at all seven categories. Use this guide to understand your scores, and to consider ways to protect your health. Your scores can change over time; check yourself again in the future to remain aware of your situation.

Numerical Ranking

A total score of 0-10: You still have a lot to discover and learn in this category. If you feel you are ready for change, you have already taken the first step towards becoming more resilient. Use materials provided throughout the chapter on Resilience to help you grow.

A total score of 11-20: You rank in the midrange in this category. If you want to improve your resilience, pick one of the statements that seem especially important to you and ask yourself the following questions:

- In what things am I successful in my life, why did I pick this number?

- What would it take to reach a higher number of points?

- How would this improve my life?

- Which actions would I have to take to achieve this?

A total score of 21-30: You are already an expert in this category! Surely you are satisfied with yourself in these areas and often experience empowering events. These are your strengths and resources and you can use them to compensate for other, weaker areas.

© **Resilience Project** (open access) http://www.resilience-project.eu/uploads/media/self_evaluation_en.pdf

Resilience Activity #2: What will I do to build my resilience?

Action Plan for Building Resilience **Directions:** Read through items on the chart. Check those that you want to "keep doing" and those you'd like to "start to do" or "do more often." If other resilience-building behaviors come to mind, write them in on the blank lines provided in each section.	Keep Doing	Start Doing Do More
Physical		
1. Exercise.		
2. Get adequate sleep and rest.		
3. Practice good hygiene and grooming; dress well.		
4. Use medicine as prescribed; limit alcohol.		
5. Avoid using drugs or tobacco.		
6.		
7.		
Nutritional		
1. Eat a balanced, healthy diet.		
2. Get and adequate intake of fluid.		
3. Avoid eating empty calories.		
4. Limit salt, saturated fat and trans fats.		
5. Snack on healthy foods.		
6.		
7.		
Medical		
1. Access quality health care.		
2. Get preventive screenings: E.g. Blood pressure, diabetes, eyes.		
3. Prevent injuries.		
4. Manage and rehab injuries that have occurred.		
5. Manage chronic health conditions.		
6.		
7.		

Action Plan for Building Resilience *Continued*	Keep Doing	Start Doing Do More
Environmental		
1. Recognize and address environmental stressors: • Temperature		
• Noise and interruptions		
• Air quality.		
2. Take measures to assure safety in my home or workplace.		
3. Take measures to prevent injuries in my home or workplace.		
4. Avoid taking unnecessary risks.		
5. Do things to organize or beautify my home or workplace.		
6.		
7.		
Psychological		
1. Think and do things to boost my confidence and self-belief.		
2. Think in optimistic ways and change pessimistic thoughts.		
3. Practice mindfulness.		
4. Use active problem-solving behavior.		
5. Identify my feelings and share my feelings with others.		
6. Persist in my efforts, even when encountering difficulty.		
7. Accept uncertainty and ambiguity.		
8. Use re-relabeling to help mentally cope with difficulties.		
9. Use physical activity to work-off intense emotions.		
10.		
11.		
12.		

Action Plan for Building Resilience *Continued*	Keep Doing	Start Doing Do More
Social		
1. Reach out to people and groups who provide positive support: Emotional, informational and/or hands-on-help.		
2. Participate in groups that offer support: In-person groups, online or telephone support groups.		
3. Try to imitate the lives and actions of inspiring individuals.		
4. Enjoy fun activities, hobbies, and socializing with others.		
5. Take time-off from doing work of any kind, and time to be alone.		
6. If employed outside the home, mentally separate work and home.		
7.		
8.		
Spiritual		
1. Identify the values, beliefs and purpose that give my life meaning.		
2. Regularly connect with God or what gives my life meaning.		
3. Regularly pray, worship or meditate.		
4. Enjoy experiences of nature or the arts.		
5. Read texts, watch shows, and listen to music that is inspiring.		
6.		
7.		

Helpful Resources

Southwick, Steven and Charney, Dennis. ***Resilience: The Science of Mastering Life's Greatest Challenges.*** Second Edition. Cambridge University Press. 2018.

Wagonild, Gail. ***True Resilience: Building a Life of Strength, Courage and Meaning. Cape House Books. 2014.*** Find additional resources at ***The Resilience Center***: https://www.resiliencecenter.com/ which presents a wide range of evidence-based materials for researchers as well as a Brief Resilience Scale for the general public.

Walsh, Froma. ***Strengthening Family Resilience.*** 3nd Edition. Guilford Press. 2016.

....

"Resilience is accepting your new reality, even if it's less good than the one you had before."
Elizabeth Edwards
American attorney, author, and healthcare activist

"When fear rushed in, I learned how to hear my heart racing but refused to allow my feelings to sway me. That resilience came from my family. It flowed through our bloodline."
Coretta Scott King
American author, activist, civil rights leader
The wife of Martin Luther King Jr.

"Do not judge me by my success, judge me by how many times I fell down and got back up again."
Nelson Mandela
Former President of South Africa

....